ENVIRONMENTS FOR HEALTH

ENVIRONMENTS FOR HEALTH

A SALUTOGENIC APPROACH

John J. Macdonald

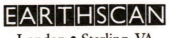

London • Sterling, VA

First published by Earthscan in the UK and USA

Copyright © John J. Macdonald

First South Asian Edition 2007

ISBN-13: 978-1-85383-476-9
ISBN-10: 1-85383-476-9
ISBN-13: 978-1-85383-477-6
ISBN-10: 1-85383-477-7

Typeset by Pantek Arts Ltd, Maidstone, Kent
Printed in India by Brijbasi Art Press Ltd., I-72, Sector-9, Noida
Cover design by Yvonne Booth

For a full list of publications please contact:

Earthscan
8-12 Camden High Street
London, NW1 0JH, UK
Tel: +44 (0)20 7387 8558
Fax: +44(0)20 7387 8998
Email: earthinfo@earthscan.co.uk
Web: www.earthscan.co.uk

22883 Quicksilver Drive, Sterling, VA 20166-2012, USA

Earthscan is an imprint of James & James (Science Publishers) Ltd and
publishes in association with the International Institute for Environment
and Development

A catalogue record for this book is available from the British Library

Library of Congress Cataloging-in-Publication Data has been applied for

Printed on elemental chlorine-free paper

CONTENTS

ACKNOWLEDGEMENTS

First of all, I need to acknowledge my publishers, Earthscan, who have not given up on me even though I changed continents and jobs and experienced a major debilitating disease between the initial discussions about this book and its completion in 2004. Specifically, thanks to Jonathan Sinclair Wilson. The person who has inspired me most in my values in health and who demonstrates many of these values in her personal and professional life is Professor Rita Giacaman, founder of the Institute of Community and Public Health of Birzeit University in Palestine, with whom I have been privileged to work for over a decade. She sees the common good as the essence of public health, and peace and justice as obvious important components, whether on a national or international scale. I dedicate the book to her. Many people should be mentioned, I can only refer to a few of them as significant contributors to my own health and sense of well-being: my sisters/friends Kathleen, Mary and Joan, my 'mates', Michael and Air Woods, Peter and Edna Blanchard, Phil and Christine Emery and their family, Fr Paul Hanna, Murielle Koks Bosch, Jacqueline Hayden, Heather Garner and Anang Ristiawan. I hope they know how much I, and therefore this book, owe to them. Along with Rita Giacaman, I make special mention of the two people whose father I am privileged to be: my daughter Mira and son Rohan, as well as their mother, Josna. Kay Powell was a tremendous help in pulling some threads of the book together: I thank her.

LIST OF ACRONYMS AND ABBREVIATIONS

ADD	attention deficiency disorder
ADHD	attention deficiency hyperactivity disorder
GNP	gross national product
HAI	hospital associated illness
PFI	Private Finance Initiative
PHC	Primary Health Care
WHO	World Health Organization

INTRODUCTION

'THE WORLD NEEDS'

'The principal characteristic of a true thinker (*un vrai intellectuel*) is humility'. These are the words of a Father Faucher, a French Canadian priest who taught me moral philosophy in the 1960s. Although I was 'no more than a boy' when I heard them, all my intuition told me he was sharing something profound; in fact, his words have been used by me throughout my life as a test of whether I was in the presence of wisdom or simply cleverness, or indeed something even less worthy, whether in academic or non-academic contexts. I took him to mean that a person on the way to wisdom is always in awe of what we as a species (and therefore he or she as an individual) do *not* know, however laden with diplomas or expert words.

In the context of human health, humility should not be that difficult to achieve. In the first instance, the intricacy of human biology, as we discover more and more of the complexity of the specific parts of the human body and their inter-linkings, should make us gasp in wonder, not simply reel off ever more complicated descriptions of what we witness in the mystery of living organisms. Add to this the enormous intricacy of human beings' mental processes, and the interconnection between these and the biological, and we are truly in the presence of 'many splendoured' and even wondrous phenomena. Examples abound: small children, well cared for by nurses and doctors, but with no access to the loving touch of adults committed to them, like parents, fail to thrive; there can be a physical (positive) reaction in the immune systems of adults with chronic illness when the person involved experiences love and support; studies in social biology indicate how the wider social world, of unemployment or of affirmative cultural support can impact significantly for good or ill on people's health.

'What the world needs' is rather a grandiose way of beginning a book, but sometimes we may have to risk the danger of the big statement and I do so now as I begin this book:

> *What the world needs in terms of health care is a new framework, a new way of thinking health, leading to a new way of planning and doing health care.*

It is a characteristic of our time that it is possible, and indeed even necessary, to identify a global culture of health care, modified by some local and political circumstances, but generally recognizable in terms of institutions of allopathic medicine staffed by western-style trained personnel and sometimes reaching out into the community. The vast proportion of cash spent on health care by governments and individuals in the world is spent on systems of health care based on this more or less westernized acute care model. The imbalance of these systems, with their overemphasis on cure, as opposed to care and prevention or maintenance of health, is well documented (Macdonald, 2000).

The problem is that, despite all their glamour and at least implicit promises to solve all the health problems of the world, such health systems are failing many, if not most, of their clients. In both 'developed' and 'developing' countries, the cracks are showing in the health system. For moral and economic reasons, as well as to achieve improved health outcomes, we need a new model, a new framework for thinking health and planning health systems. The 20th century witnessed at least one considerable movement in this direction, fostered by the World Health Organization (WHO), the outlines of which were contained in the 'Health for All' or Primary Health Care (PHC) movement. For a variety of reasons that will be touched on, this movement did not have the impact its advocates, present writer included, had intended. Some attention is paid to the rise and fall of PHC in this book, simply because the ideals it sought to pursue, the critique of biomedicine it contained and the broad policies it envisaged are still relevant and the lessons of that time are still to be learned.

There are some indications that we as a global culture are moving, however slowly, towards a new model, a new way of thinking and of seeing health and health care. The speed of this movement has to be accelerated. This book sets out to chart the main steps of this movement and to indicate some of the ways of thinking and action that can help form new ways of approaching health care. It is hoped that the book can contribute in a modest way to the creation of more rational, just and balanced health care systems.

Chapter 1 deals with the framework we need to transcend. Chapter 2 traces the historical efforts, notably those inspired by the WHO, to grow beyond the limitations of the narrow framework of western medicine. Chapter 3 deals with the new insights and the new force of argument that are becoming available to help widen our perspectives on health and health care, specifically through the work on the social determinants of health. Chapter 4 points towards other health cultures, which reinforce and can inspire an emerging global model. Chapter 5 attempts to delineate the outlines of this expanded model, which we can call a salutogenic health framework. Finally, Chapter 6 illustrates the approach using the example of one subsection of the community often overlooked: men and their health.

John J. Macdonald

I

STILL IN THE BUSINESS OF FIXING UP

We medical men are wayside repairers of the human machines which break down on the road of life.

Sir A. Keith, *The Engines of the Human Body*

Mammy ... she used tae always go tae auld Doctor McKillop, who's aboot ninety-three and gies ye Sudofed tablets whether you've a broken leg or a broken hert.

Anne Donovan, *Buddha Da*

One of the major tasks of the postgraduate training of doctors and nurses is to re-humanise the practice of medicine.

Professor Rita Giacaman, Birzeit University, Palestine

THE MEDICAL MODEL: AN ENDURING IMBALANCED VISION AND PRACTICE

Depending on one's point of view, western medicine is either at a peak of great achievement or going through a time of serious crisis. Either way, the key is technology and the role one attributes to it. On the one hand, there have been vast developments in the area of medical technology, which have led, among other things, to the development of genetic medicine, with the promise held out of eliminating all disease. This can be seen as incredible progress, the human mind reaching out to fend off menacing influences of disease and to enhance our lives and health as never before imaginable. Others would see that this emphasis on biological manipulation is part of a fundamental and ever deepening illusion, and that a dependence on scientific technology will never 'cure the world's ills'. The most striking example is perhaps that given by the HIV/AIDS epidemic, claiming some 3 million lives in 2002 alone

(UNAIDS, 2002). Technology alone was never going to 'solve' the problems associated with the management of this condition and the healing of the individuals and communities afflicted by it. The vast amounts of money spent on this approach (looking to technical solutions) to the neglect of the care of those families affected by the epidemic is a striking example of how distorted our thinking and policies can get by pursuing the notion of technical solutions to human problems.

There are those who see the current crisis of medicine as one of funding: there never seems to be enough money to meet everyone's 'health' needs, even in the most advanced economies. It is not difficult to persuade the general public that more money for some new medical technology or for more hospital beds is an 'urgent necessity'. In some countries, the road to election time is scattered with promises of new hospitals, or at least new hospital beds. Health professionals and others working on behalf of a better distribution of health resources in support of health initiatives in the community are wary of imminent elections since these can tempt politicians to promise more technical medicine (buildings, beds, machines) and the personnel to staff them, almost inevitably taking money away from the less glamorous work of sustaining health in the community. The assumption here is that we have got it right really, this business of health – we have the right road map, all that is needed is to throw more money at it.

Others would see health systems undergoing a crisis of *credibility*. People are losing faith in health systems. To be fair, this is sometimes due to unrealistic expectations: in a world in which there is an implicit assumption of the possibility of perfect health, by which is meant the total absence of disease, discontent is inbuilt. The inevitability of some forms of suffering – and death itself – is something often absent from public consciousness in modern global culture.

Large amounts of gross national product (GNP) are spent on health systems: US 13.6 per cent, UK 8.2 per cent, Australia 9.8 per cent (Brown, 2004; National Health Debate and Poll, 2004). Despite this considerable spending, many people are discontent with health services. There is the embarrassment of iatrogenesis and hospital associated illness (HAI): conditions which people didn't have when they went into care, but picked up during their stay in the institution or other contact with the health care system. It is often only the necessity of publishing plans to reduce the number of these conditions that has given this phenomenon some publicity in recent years. There is increasing documentation of the rise in the extent of drug-resistant conditions, often due to an over-prescription of antibiotics. Solutions based on technology seem to be failing.

DISCONTENT: PEOPLE VOTING WITH THEIR FEET, 'COMPLEMENTARY MEDICINE'

In many industrialized countries, people are seeking help from 'alternative' or 'complementary' therapies. This last nomenclature is often an inaccurate description of the relationship between systems, since in many cases both 'allopathic' and 'alternative' therapists do *not* see one another as 'complementing' the skills and insights of the other, but rather as the holders of different views, competitors both in terms of ideas and for patients' loyalty and payments. The uptake in western societies of the services of naturopaths, homeopaths, spiritual healers and other non-conventional practitioners is a clear indication of population dissatisfaction with conventional health care and of the need for a major rethink for conventional, 'allopathic' health services. People are voting with their feet and, importantly, with their purses and wallets. Talking of this situation, Ernst has this to say:

> *In essence, therefore, no single determinant of the present popularity of complementary and alternative medicine exists, but there is a broad range of interacting positive and negative motivations. Some of these amount to a biting criticism of our modern healthcare system. Regardless of whether this criticism is valid or not, it is often deeply felt by those who turn towards complementary and alternative medicine, and mainstream medicine would be well advised to consider it seriously.*
>
> Ernst (2000), p1133

In a broad global perspective, colonization by western countries has involved a process of cultural colonization or imperialism, whereby colonized people have often come to see themselves and their culture, including their healing systems, through the eyes of the colonizers (Fanon, 1968). The result has been a massive underdevelopment of traditional medicines and the wholehearted adoption by many of the values and approach of western medicine. The great irony here is that in the west, the discontent with allopathic medicine to which we have referred has grown and brought about, in the west itself, not only a keen interest in but wide-scale practice of non-western medicines, as well as extensive growth of 'alternative' or 'complementary' therapies. Perhaps the most striking example lies with Chinese traditional medicine; in particular, the practice of acupuncture. Twenty years ago this practice was widely described in the west as dangerous nonsense. Now it is not only widely accepted, with westerners seeking out Chinese practitioners, but many western doctors are following courses in acupuncture techniques. This is extremely interesting from the point of view of philosophy, notably the philosophy of science, since western medicine cannot justify acupuncture within the limits of its own parameters. The 'meridians' or mediators of the energy flows, which explain the practice of acupuncture and acupressure, are not susceptible to scientific observation as western science knows it. The practice is established, often 'justified' in western scientific terms, but in fact represents a real challenge to the parameters of thought of western medical science. The real irony, of course, lies in the phenomenon of 'developing' countries, having been brainwashed to reject traditional healing systems as backward and unscientific, now witnessing not only the adoption of many of these practices by western societies, but even endorsement by international agencies. The very processes of global colonization that undermined traditional medicine in the first place will now endorse its reintroduction into developing countries, of course modified and commercialized even more than it was in the past.

DISTINGUISHING THE BABY FROM THE BATH WATER

The baby

There can be no denying the great achievements of western medicine and the progress it has made in terms of recognizing and dealing with some major human conditions of disease. Those of us who have criticized the 'medical model' must nevertheless (humbly) acknowledge all the genuine alleviation of human suffering that has been achieved through certain practices of western health systems; in the context of older people's health it has been pointed out that:

> *The power of medical care to improve the quality of life should not be disregarded. Surgery for things such as hernias, cataracts, prostate, varicose veins and hip joints may not be glamorous or do very much to improve life expectancy, but they are important to the quality of life of old people.*
>
> Blane et al (1995), p11

And in a wider global perspective, the WHO is right to remind us of the considerable achievements involved in the eradication of smallpox and the reduced risk to millions of people of infectious diseases such as yellow fever, poliomyelitis, measles and diphtheria (WHO, 2002a).

The bath water

Such achievements notwithstanding, the western model of health care is, at the very least, straining within the expectations put upon it, or that it puts upon itself. What it seems to lack, despite the lessons that are there to be learned about its limitations, is humility. The assumption seems to be that only time and money are needed to ensure that in the development of technologies we will find all the answers to the health issues of the world. Medicine will conquer all. This optimism, however, has created a tension within western popular culture and within the profession itself. Sickness and disease seem as much part of individual and collective life as ever. People still fall sick, age and die. Doctors are understandably frustrated by the expectations of cure put upon them by society; many people in western societies having been brought up to turn to the medical profession when healing of any sort is required. The role of the doctor as priest and spiritual comforter in a secular society is readily observable, a reality not necessarily pursued by the medical profession but one thrust upon them by a needy population (Bauer, 2001).

BEYOND MEDICINE

Not all conditions of illness can be cured, and certainly not all from within the repertoire of the healing tools available to the average doctor, nurse or hospital. Much of the causes of disease lie outside the control of the health profession, as do, likewise, much of the well-springs of health and healing. They lie, in general terms, in the context of people's lives. The idea of the importance of *context*, environment or life circumstances has long been recognized in public health in, for example, the use of the analogy of 'upstream', 'downstream'. Some doctors, nurses and other health workers realize that they are often busy with the symptoms of problems. As a result, they are frequently dealing with 'downstream': populations, people who have fallen into the 'river of illness', while being conscious that 'upstream' – in the wider social context of people's lives – lie the causes of much illness, whether in the personal, social or economic domain. The idea of 'specific aetiology' of disease (one sickness with one cause, the latter to be identified and eliminated) is generally seen as so simplistic as to be of no account (Macdonald, 2000) even if this approach still influences some medical practice.

THE NEED FOR NEW VISION

The emphasis on technical competence to deal with pathologies, often within institutions of expensive treatment, almost always takes precedence over any attempt to argue for a broader view and vision involving a community-based focus and community-based mechanisms, which deal with local issues and working links and access to systems 'higher up'. The need for such mechanisms and such an approach is increasingly being felt in both developing and developed countries:

> *Across a whole continent – Africa – our age is witness to the tragedy of an epidemic of unimaginable proportions. At the end of 2002 there were 42 million people living with HIV/AIDS, of whom 29.4 million in sub-Saharan Africa.*
>
> UNAIDS (2002)

The disappearance of a whole generation, those we can describe in economic terms as 'productive': men and women aged 18–45, has meant that top-down health services, often hospital based, even with the best will in the world, are left standing impotent in the face of the health needs not only of patients but, just as tragically, their children and the older generation left to care for them. Similar tragic scenarios are emerging in other continents. It is not simply that health systems have not been able to cope, it is rather that the health systems, following a globalized notion of health care, using whatever finances they have mainly on hospitals and acute care – by and large for those who can afford these – have been shown to be imbalanced and flawed in their basic assumptions and approach. Where logic would call for great effort at prevention and early intervention as community based as possible, the structures (and often mentalities) in place are focused on disease in hospitals.

The same imbalance shows as much in so-called developed countries where we have the phenomenon of an ageing population and a health system often geared to acute rather than chronic care, often missing the needs of this population in a serious way.

> *Today, one of every 10 persons is 60 years old or over, totalling 629 million people worldwide. By 2050, the United Nations projects that one of every five persons will be 60 or older, and that by 2150 this ratio will be one of every three persons. By 2050, the actual number of people over the age of 60 is projected to be almost 2 billion, at which point the population of older persons will outnumber children (0–14 years).*
> United Nations (2002), Article 2

Being old is not an illness, nor does it necessarily involve illness. But there is no doubt that many older people, one may say, *naturally* experience some form of chronic illness as life progresses. The management of this situation in an efficient and humane way is an enormous challenge for society at large and health services in particular. Again we see the serious flaws in a system focusing largely on acute care: a hospital-based system which, given the high cost of modern technology and health professionals, consumes the greatest proportion of the health budget to the detriment of many older people who are in need of another approach to care that is less institution based and addresses their needs for treatment and maintenance of health *where they live* or as close to it as possible. Of course, ageing is also a phenomenon challenging health systems worldwide and not just in developed countries, as is witnessed by the recent WHO initiative of an integrated response to 'rapid population ageing' (WHO, undated, Ageing and Life Course Program).

Health systems in poorer countries with hospitals overflowing with children who are suffering from preventable illnesses or dying from conditions for which their families cannot afford treatment or which are amenable to community-based solutions if identified early, are facing an imbalance similar to that in the health systems of 'richer' countries with hospitals containing large cohorts of elderly patients suffering from chronic conditions, often with a 'psychosomatic' dimension, who could be cared for outside the hospital and often in their own homes. The problem is basically the same in both situations: we are using the wrong tools for the job, investing in a lopsided 'health' system: medicine has 'its place' in the rational planning of the provision of care, but expecting medicine to 'create' and maintain health and prevent disease is clearly asking too much of it. Hospital-based systems cannot provide the panacea many still expect them to. But we will not creatively expand and develop our health systems unless there is a popular and professional development of thinking around health and health systems. We need another way to *think* health and *do* health care.

HEALTH OUT OF CONTEXT

The above scenario of mismatch between 'problem' and 'solution', whether in the paediatric or HIV/AIDS wards of the developing world or the general or geriatric wards of hospitals in industrialized countries, encapsulates an important dimension of the crisis of modern medicine: an individual doctor or nurse faced with a collection of individual patients. The 'causes' of the conditions presented by the patients often lie, at least partially, in the social, economic, cultural and personal emotional and spiritual *context* or environment of the patients. On discharge, the patients will return to their living environment, which will either foster or hinder their healing, help to maintain them in health or precipitate them again towards illness. Yet the health professional and the patient are meeting in an individualized medical situation in which the pressure is for the professional to 'fix things up', to provide a total 'cure'. The whole therapeutic encounter tends to be decontextualized.

Individual engineering

This model of 'dramatic' health care in which the health professional, generally a doctor, diagnoses what is wrong with an individual patient, perceived as a free-floating decontextualized individual, and prescribes treatment, whether chemical or surgical, with its underpinning framework of the specialist fixing up a broken-down machine, has outlived its usefulness yet it still underpins both much of health care practice and public expectation of health systems throughout the world. It is this model which has been globalized.

The reductionism involved when systems and the attitudes formed by them are built on this framework of 'mending the broken-down individual machine' cannot be underestimated in terms of its harmful effects, not only as regards the decontextualization and so dehumanization of the healing process, but also with regard to the effectiveness of that process.

As for decontextualization: take off a person's clothes, put them in a hospital or surgical slip – removed from their family, their loved ones, their culture, their familiar world and a great deal of themselves is removed. As the saying has it: 'I am me and my circumstances'. Many have pointed to the dangers involved in the Cartesian legacy in western thought whereby the human being is conceived of as a body/machine somehow inhabited by a spirit, body and mind being almost separate entities or at least well-differentiated compartments of a machine. It is this individualized broken-down machine which is the focus of the medical 'gaze'; this is what is seen, the object of medical attention. There is much evidence to challenge this way of thinking. Body and mind are more linked than we ever imagined and the body-mind of the person is largely a product of and dependent on the total environment in which he/she lives, being nourished or diminished by the material and spiritual world in which they are immersed and in which life is lived out. A point to be made here is that, unless we actively pursue other analogies, other ways of seeing the human reality than the decontextualized body-mind individual-machine, it is very likely that we will continue to practise medicine and plan services in ways informed by this reductionist dualism. We need new ways of thinking and doing 'health'. We need to think of health in a much more whole or holistic contextualized way and in the light of this rearrange our services accordingly.

THE CARTESIAN DEBT

Western medicine owes a great debt to the analogy of the body as a machine. The concept helped European culture move away from a magical view of health and illness which, at its worst, left people at the whim of nature, evil spirits, or God:

> *As flies to wanton boys, are we to the Gods*
> *They kill us for their sport.*
>
> Shakespeare, *King Lear*

The drive to understand 'what is happening' in human organisms, inspired by Descartes, has moved us away from this fatalistic passive attitude whereby human beings are potential victims of chance. Following the insights of western philosophy, inspired by scholars such as Descartes, the processes of healing became more organized in terms of critical examination of the human body and its functioning or malfunctioning: no longer subject to random acts of fate or unkindly spirits or vapours, and capable of rational explanation. Other societies had for many centuries critically observed the interaction between the person and their environment, notably the world of herbs and plants and even the social and built environment. The Cartesian suggestion that the body is like a machine – a clock for instance – and the subsequent dissection of human cadavers bringing a greater understanding of the internal functioning of some of the individual organs of the body, tended, however, in the western tradition, to remove context from the picture. Great progress was made in the human understanding of the part of illness which is represented by the malfunctioning of body systems. But this process of reduction, isolating the component parts in order to understand them better, almost inevitably loses sight of the whole. 'The sum is greater than the parts' is a truism but nonetheless relevant in this case: the human being is more than the sum of its body parts; human health is more than the efficient functioning of these parts. We can say that the human existence is largely a contextualized one and it is often in the context of people's lives that lie the roots both of their ill health and their well-being.

ATTACKING ILLNESS

This reductionist tendency in western medicine has been combined with a rather arrogant attitude towards healing, conceptualizing it as the result of the imposition of the rational mind over nature: through the mastery of science, through understanding the mechanics of living organisms, human beings would be able to 'conquer' sickness by interventions aimed at arresting harmful processes. It is fair to describe western medicine in this sense as 'aggressive' (Kaptchuk, 2000). Some humility would have been and still is useful; for example, some acknowledgement of the agency of the body itself, the energy within each human being that interacts with the environment it finds itself in. Even interventions such as antibiotics and surgery are procedures that remove obstacles from the path the body will follow in order to heal itself. This is not often acknowledged, let alone 'understood', in the training of western health practitioners. There is a deal of arrogance, which persists, for example, in the claims of modern genetic medicine to 'cure all illness', a matter to which we shall return. At its most bellicose, western scientific medicine trumpets its 'total' control of the natural processes of illness and healing, if not as something yet possessed and mastered, at least as something attainable in the foreseeable future. The fact is, however, that this model no longer fits what we now know of the complexities, both of the human body and of the genesis of health and illness.

THE UNACKNOWLEDGED: THE HUMAN LIFE FORCE
ENGAGING WITH ITS ENVIRONMENT

Machines do not heal; living persons heal, what we could call their *life force* reasserts itself, seeking to find a renewed balance with its environment. The true healer, in any culture, is the respectful witness and attendant of this process. Midwifery as a profession has in many cases learned this lesson of humility, though we witness in our day the tension between the focus on 'attending' the natural processes of birth and a focus on intervention to preclude the possibility of danger. This notion of health as essentially a dynamic process of the human being interacting with his/her environment seems at once too simple and too complex for the western mind to grasp easily. It is indeed much easier to think of health as the absence of disease and the task of the healer to be the removal of what is going wrong in the functioning of the human body.

In a western society, a young, socially isolated mother goes to the doctor, feeling 'run down'. She is short of cash, is bringing up three children on her own in public housing and smokes several packets of cigarettes a day. She is on antidepressants – technical medical interventions. Her eldest child, a boy, has always been 'difficult to handle' and, after consultation between the boy's teacher, the doctor and the anxious mother, has been receiving medication for attention deficiency hyperactivity disorder (ADHD) for some years now. So there are at least two members of the family being 'healed' or at least helped to maintain their health by the system. Such a scenario, give or take some variations, is very common in many western countries. The doctor knows that the smoking is a coping mechanism for this mother, knows also the inadequacy of the intervention that medicine can offer: a repeat prescription for the antidepressant, the suggestion of nicotine patches, and a gentle reminder of the damaging effect of the cigarette smoking on her and the children's health as well as the expression of hope that the behavioural patterns of the child which are diagnosed as an illness will disappear in time. The doctor's experience tells him or her that the context of these two patients' lives is an essential component of their health and often has a vague realization that some improvements in the interaction between the family and their environment must feature largely in any healing 'plan'. But what can the doctor do, more than the simple interventions suggested? Health has become a decontextualized technical business.

In industrialized countries, a large percentage of falls of older people resulting in hospitalization occur in their homes when they are on their own and experiencing the disorientation that can come with social isolation. As a result of the fall, they enter the world of 'health' (actually, the *disease* system). The hospital system spends time and money on the consequences of this and many other preventable conditions, just as much as the hospitals in developing countries find themselves dealing with malnourished children who, much more cheaply and effectively, could have been 'rehabilitated' closer to their home and have been prevented from being malnourished in the first place. Many creative initiatives of what the Third World knows as 'Primary Health Care' have arisen from the realization of the necessity to deal with context as well as treating individuals, handling the downstream victims as well as working hard with communities upstream to prevent them falling into the river of illness in the first place.

All these situations – malnourished hospitalized children, the isolated young mother and the falls of older people – point to the inadequacies of a health system geared mainly to addressing individual pathology in institutions of care rather than spending time and money dealing with prevention and localized, appropriate care in the community. In theory, some medical practitioners might say that, sure, more money is needed for community health work, but evidence suggests that while we retain present mindsets the terrible imbalance will remain largely unchallenged.

THE MEDICAL ENGINEERING MODEL MINDSET

It is a terrible caricature of the biomedical model to see the institution of care as a garage, the doctor as a mechanic and the patient as a broken-down car. But, as with many caricatures, there are elements of truth embedded in it. Western medicine *does* tend to reduce what is complex in health and illness to the aggressive elimination/correction of something that is wrong with the patient by some sort of chemical or surgical intervention. Moreover, as a health system, it *does* tend to be reactive in operation, waiting for something to go wrong and then intervening: the focus is on dealing with the crisis of the pathological rather than the building up of health. This has been called the 'fire-engine' approach: the system waits for the flames to break out then sends out a fire engine to deal with it. The model also focuses on the professional doing something *for* the sick person rather than *in partnership with* the patient. Most of all, perhaps, as has been said, 'scientific medicine' tends to decontextualize the phenomenon of ill health, to see it in isolation from the environment in which the person who is ill lives: by this is meant, of course, not only the physical environment, essential though this is, but also the social, emotional, psychological, spiritual and economic environment of the presenting person. The patient is conceived as being in a passive role, and the dynamic in which the professional is active and the patient passive tends to be the norm in this globalized culture of health care. Individual 'patients' and committed health professionals may squirm at the caricature elements of this model but there can be little doubt that, as a picture, it accurately reflects how health systems are generally organized. Circumstances combine to ensure the survival of this framework of reference, in which health care systems see the process of healing as the domain of professionals who are paid to fix the machine after it gets broken. And this way of 'thinking health and doing health care' is alive and well in both popular and professional health cultures throughout the world.

If we look to 'western popular health culture', the way people are influenced by the globalized approach to health systems originating in western societies, one can observe the tendency to look for the 'quick fix' of medicine. The medical profession, despite protests to the contrary, is still linked to its image as purveyor of the *magic bullet*. Antibiotics have done much to keep alive the mindset which sees the health system in terms of 'fix-it up' medical mechanics. And antibiotics stand as a potent symbol of the imbalances that can result from this reductionist approach that has shaped western medicine:

Resistance [to antibiotics] is not a new phenomenon: it was recognized early as a scientific curiosity and then as a threat to effective treatment outcome. However, the development of new families of antimicrobials throughout the 1950s and 1960s and of modifications of these molecules through the 1970s and 1980s allowed us to believe that we could always remain ahead of the pathogens. By the turn of the century this complacency had come to haunt us. The pipeline of new drugs is running dry and the incentives to develop new antimicrobials to address the global problems of drug resistance are weak.

WHO (2001), p1

It is antibiotics or some other quick-fix intervention that Miss Polly perhaps looked for and certainly obtained when she 'sent for the doctor':

> *Miss Polly had a dolly who was sick, sick, sick*
> *So she called for the doctor to come quick, quick, quick*
> *The doctor came with his bag and his hat*
> *And he knocked on the door with a rat-a-tat-tat*
> *He looked at the dolly and he shook his head*
> *He said, 'Miss Polly put her straight to bed'*
> *He wrote on a paper for a pill, pill, pill,*
> *And said, 'I'll be back in the morning with my bill, bill, bill'.*

Nursery rhymes sometimes reflect deeply held cultural beliefs; in this case, of the nature of a reactive, quick-fix, profession-led and commodified health system.

DIFFERING PERCEPTIONS OF THE 'PROBLEM'

International and national reports call for reform of the health system, though often from completely different points of view.

'The problem is lack of resources'

There are calls for more money to do more of the same: more cash, it is regularly argued, would mean that health care systems would have shorter waiting lists for surgery, better cardiac surgery outcomes and so forth. In newspapers throughout the industrialized world, journalists in search of a 'good health story' have only to attend any accident and emergency unit or other area of dramatic medicine to acquire a story of the lack of resources, sometimes human, but often material: beds and medical technology. Already, health care systems are consuming more and more of national budgets, allocated disproportionately towards hospital treatment and medical, profession-based technical interventions like surgery and drug-based therapies. Such scenarios, we have said, are the stuff of pre-election political campaigns. Any attempt to raise a voice for a greater balance between prevention and cure in the system, between community care and acute care, gets lost in the clamour for the 'right' to the best medical technology *now*.

What is urgently required is a culture in which a more enlightened public and profession will think *health* and not just the dramatic treatment of disease. This is not just a plea for a systems approach to health care. It is also a call for a more holistically trained medical profession who can see upstream and downstream in whatever section of the system they work. It is a call for 'health-promoting public health policies' to provide the cultural and material base on which the health of individuals and communities can be built. But, in addition, it is a call for a genuine public education, a more informed citizenry which will give more weight than at present to the preventive and promotive wings of health care. Unless there is such a double-pronged educational initiative, it is unlikely that we will soon be focusing our attention and resources 'upstream'.

'We are not sufficiently business oriented in medicine'

Another strand of opinion has it that a main problem has been the failure to embrace the fact that medicine is a business and must take its place in the market economy, unashamedly. This latter view is clearly the one espoused as a global recipe by the World Bank in its prescription for better health and health care, as we can see in such documents as the World Bank Annual Report of 1993 entitled *Investing in Health*. Much of the language of health *outcomes* and health *gain* is underpinned by this way of thinking, even if the rationale is not often explicit. Cost effectiveness is the major criterion of success and informs much of the thinking about many so-called health reforms: can we get more measurable outcomes from the same health dollar? Part of the problem here is that an understandable profit motive – medicine as a well-paid career and medical systems as profitable enterprises – as well as the perfectly laudable aim of efficiency are combined with a rhetoric of service and community good. Some more honest realism may be called for. 'Ethics' in medical education rarely deals with macro-morality, for example, the moral dimension of significant numbers of national populations being excluded on account of poverty from access to decent medical services – if we invest in this or that particular technology, then there will be less for the care of the elderly, for those not able to pay full whack. In this context, it is significant that as long ago as 1990 it was noted that 31 million Americans had no access to primary care (Garrett, 2000, p558). Others would put the figure closer to 40 million. Technical medicine is increasingly perceived as a commodity to be bought: the voice of the tradition that held that health and the means to achieve it are a human right grows faint and even begins to sound like an historical semi-religious statement of belief. The market economy has come to dominate our global culture, with obvious impact on health care.

One of the contradictions emerging in the issues to do with the market economy's increasing dominance of health care is one illustrated by the Private Finance Initiative (PFI) in the UK.

> The [UK] government hands control of new public works to a private consortium. The financiers borrow the money to build a hospital ... the consortium rents it to the NHS (National Health System) for 30–60 years ... the consortium must make a profit.
>
> Cohen (2004)

This has led to the owners restricting hospital intakes which are not profitable, a sad case of the only effective restraint on the 'medical model' being economic rationalism.

Calls for more money for action in the acute activities of any system are often strident, fuelled, as we have said, both by popular culture's belief in dramatic medicine and the medical profession's need for the latest technology. With such a dominant 'discourse', there is not much chance of people listening to the voice that calls for resources for prevention and for humble and unromantic work like the assurance of a supportive environment for isolated elderly and young families, and for community-based support systems for persons with HIV/AIDS and their families.

'We have lost the health plot'

There are, of course, voices that have been saying for some decades now that global health systems, inspired by western health care, have lost their way, not because they are not receiving sufficient funding, or making enough money, but precisely because the financial incentive taken to extreme distorts the whole picture, that the *moral* dimension to the management of health is being lost. Certainly, there is much discontent among populations.

> *In the five health care systems studied here, the views of the public appear quite similar. In no nation is a majority content with the health care system. In the United States and the United Kingdom the same concerns have persisted for a decade, and public support is largely unchanged. In Australia and, most notably, Canada, the public's confidence has been shaken. In New Zealand, where we conducted this type of survey for the first time, it is apparent that something has gone wrong and the public is anxious.*
>
> Donelan et al (1999), p213

Medicine and its great allies, the pharmaceutical companies, suggest that all that is needed is more of the same, at whatever cost. Yet many voices, both lay and professional, are being raised in protest. As Julius Nyerere of Tanzania said about the education system that African countries inherited from their colonial past: what is needed is not *more of the same* but something *completely different*. We need to gather together all those voices that are asking for another way of thinking and doing health care; a way that is both effective in meeting the health needs of the majority of populations and efficient, making the best use of the technology affordable by that society. To do this we need a way of conceptualizing health and health systems that binds the preventative and the curative into one vision and one operational system.

The challenges posed to health care systems throughout the world by such critiques as those put forward by the Alma Ata Conference (WHO, 1978) and the Primary Health Care movement are just as relevant at the beginning of the 21st century as they were in the year of the Conference in 1978 (Macdonald, 2000) (see Chapter 2 for a fuller discussion of this history).

THE NEED FOR NEW THINKING

To sum up, the challenge, or a major thrust of it, can be expressed in the following way: globalized medicine has made and continues to make great technical strides but there is an obvious imbalance in systems that put their money and status into acute care to the neglect of prevention and promotion of health and well-being. The focus, in such distorted systems, is still largely reductionist: it deals with the individual's pathologies out of context from their environment. This present book explores ways in which the principles of a new, more balanced approach can take new meaning in the light of the growing body of knowledge concerning the social determinants of health and help the general public and the medical profession think of health more as *dealing with – and enhancement of – the environment.*

'Medicine in its place': this is the subtitle of the book I wrote in 1992–93 about Primary Health Care. The words were intended to imply that medical systems do have an important place in any modern health care system. But the phrase 'medicine in its place' was also meant to advocate a better balance and to call for necessary adjustments: medicine's place in the health system needed looking at. Left to themselves, national health care systems have a tendency to favour medical technical interventions at the expense of preventive dimensions of health systems and those initiatives and procedures that are aimed at promoting the *well-being* of individuals and communities. There was nothing startlingly new in the book and its endorsement of the need for a balance between prevention and treatment; there was nothing surprising for many health workers in such a call, especially for those working on the preventative, health-promotional side of the professional spectrum. Nevertheless, by the first decade of the 21st century, we find that there is often no better balance between cure and health promotion. On the contrary, the amazing advances in technical medicine, for example, in terms of genetic medicine, still capture headlines and funding and ensure further delays in the pursuit of rational and more balanced health systems.

Genetic medicine gives new life to the medical model and hinders
progress towards a greater balance

This would be a suitable headline for a newspaper report on the contribution genetic medicine is making to the perpetuation of a culture of 'a pill for every ill'. It is not, however, one that anyone is likely to read. The media love the romance of technical medicine and its promises: they feed our collective belief in the miracle of modern science, however disappointing that promise has so far been. Newspapers loved to assure us at the turn of the 20th century that commercial companies were working to put

> *a whole genome-full of genetic sequences on a single silicon chip. [As*
> *a result] one day we might each carry with us exactly such a chip*
> *from which the doctor's computer can read any gene the better to tai-*
> *lor out prescriptions to us.*
>
> Ridley (1999), p267

Fairly typical of the media's support for this optimism is this piece from a commentator:

> **'Book of Life' promises great advances for 21st century**
> **medicine**
> *With the announcement that the entire genetic code has been*
> *mapped, scientists now have a thrilling 'to do' list for the 21st centu-*
> *ry. The goal ... is to identify and place into proper order the 3.12 bil-*
> *lion chemical base pairs present in the human DNA and to identify*
> *within that DNA the thousand of human genes ... In the near term,*
> *the new information is expected to revolutionise drug development,*
> *making it much easier for pharmaceutical companies to target their*
> *products at the* actual causes of disease. *(emphasis added)*
>
> Crenson (2000)

Although expressed in journalistic terms, the tone of the above remarks reflects fairly accurately a global tendency. The 'rat-a-tat-tat' of the doctor is heard again at the door and his bill this time will be gigantic. Faced with the splendid challenge of the 'Book of Life' and its promise of 'cure' for so many of the world's diseases by attacking the 'actual causes of disease', what is the advocate of non-romantic, non-prestigious, non-photogenic interventions of preventive medicine to do? As the Nuffield Council on Bioethics, in a report on genetic medicine and mental health, acknowledged: there is a danger that our modern interest in genetics will encourage the idea that genetic influences are of paramount importance and neglect social and other causes of illness (Caldicott et al, 1998). Given the choice, for example, on the one hand, between funding either a national programme to visit the elderly in their homes to ensure that their sense of self and well-being is sustained, or funding a sustained programme of support for the well-being of those millions of African people who support the children of parents who have died of AIDS or, on the other hand, of funding a piece of the high-tech action of the 'Book of Life' to do with genetic manipulation (for example, to 'eliminate cancer'), what government is going to fund visiting old people in their homes or carers of AIDS orphans? What National Medical Association is going to put its weight behind such initiatives if it means – as mean it must, since cash is a finite commodity – redistributing money away from some high-tech interventions and those who are the engineers of such interventions? And, just as importantly, is the tragedy not that such a disproportionate status of the new (expensive) magic bullets of scientific medicine is awarded to it not just by many members of the medical profession, but by many members of the public who, whatever their need for prevention and health promotion, have been confirmed so steadfastly in the belief in the magic bullet and the supremacy of technical medicine that they would also support such an allocation of funds? As we have said, one of the greatest needs is for popular education. Television, the great persuader, if not the great educator, regularly underpins the heroic image of technical medicine: tragic death averted by the timely intervention of high-tech medicine wielded by knowing and sympathetic doctors. The cost of such technology and the salaries of those who wield it are rarely the focus. Nor, of course, is the fate of the millions sleeping in the streets and excluded from the benefits of such health systems, even in the USA, which is the home of many of these images.

It is good to note and important to publicize examples that run counter to these tendencies – for example, the overemphasis in the 'medical model' on institutional care. The Scottish Parliament has, early in its history in the 21st century, ensured that all older people have right of access to care, regardless of their economic status (Barrow, 2004). Television is mentioned to draw attention to what is meant by the need for popular education: the big ask is for a cultural shift, a sea change in the way we think and do health and health care. The challenge is not simply to announce the need for such a change but to begin to map it out. A focus on the context of people's lives seems an essential element of such a mapping exercise and will be returned to throughout this book.

THE ENEMY WITHIN

One finds poor families in cities of industrialized countries of the north with insufficient funds for heating through the winter, and inhabitants of cities of poorer countries in the south with not enough money for children's school fees. In both contexts, I have witnessed such families take money from their stretched family budgets to contribute to yet another piece of 'latest' technical medical equipment for a cancer unit in a large hospital, where 'common sense' would dictate that such large funds be spent on prevention, if not of cancer, at least of some of the other debilitating conditions with their origins in the *context* of people's lives which afflict the populations of these places, through healthier environments, housing and the like. In some Asian and African countries we can witness the plight of committed professionals and community activists struggling to find even modest funds to ensure essential community-based health structures, for example to permit access to services by AIDS-affected families or even children with diarrhoea, having to come to terms with the ease with which public figures gain popular support by founding medical institutions such as cancer hospitals (in themselves no bad thing). I have seen the very poor, living in urban environments of the worst kind, without decent housing, transport, vying among themselves to contribute to the hero's hospital plans, in some far city or suburb. The sooner such public figures are 'converted' to the cause of *health as environment* the better. It is relatively easy to find champions of dramatic technical medical interventions, such as screening machines for children's cancer wards. It is more difficult to find stars who will put their energy behind affordable sanitation for marginalized populations in our teeming mega-cities or improvements in the housing of the post-industrial cities in the west. Yet it requires little science to indicate the enormously greater benefit of these 'health' rather than 'medical' interventions in terms of the reduction of human suffering and disease.

One would not wish in any way to challenge the generosity of such giving: I merely point to the seductive force of the medical model and to the need for a change in culture. Stakeholders such as governments, medical authorities and training establishments as well as the corporate world, have much to address in this regard.

Popular culture, supported by medicine and vested interests, encourages the public to continue to think of specialized (and again costly) technical interventions as constituting the 'real thing' in health care with everything else as poor relatives. Arguments for a more 'whole' view of health systems *can* impinge on popular consciousness but such popular health education takes time, commitment and, most of all, consistent public policies. Sometimes the issues concerning environment and health are writ larger in countries with great extremes of wealth and poverty. The huge shanty towns of the Third World are becoming more and more difficult to ignore. In many contexts, when official attention does get turned to the domain of prevention and 'health promotion', the reductionist tendency still prevails: the dominant model, in practice if not in theory, often consists of information from experts as to what the individual should or should not do, behavioural modification, rather than on the creation of health-enhancing environments. We get life-*style* health education, rather than life-*context* health education (Macdonald, 2000). We are far from a popular or professional preoccupation with health as environment, far from a contextualized view of health, far from the culture of general practitioners or other clinical practitioners with what has been called a 'public health mindset' (Watt, 2001).

THE ENEMY WITHOUT

Exhortations to people to adopt healthy lifestyles are easy and often of dubious efficacy. Frequently their focus on the individual can deflect attention from structural issues underlying problems. The journalist, George Monbiot (2001, p23), in a critique of the UK government's 'Cancer Plan' says:

> ... it contains plenty of helpful advice on giving up smoking. It outlines a scheme for increasing the amount of fruit and vegetables that children can eat. But only one pollutant is mentioned as a possible cause of cancer: radon gas, which occurs naturally.

Monbiot is making a plea that systems should acknowledge and tackle the non-personal, i.e. society-caused, origins of cancer in the *environment*. I see this as a plea for the kind of common sense and rationality that is needed for us to create new ways of thinking about health and health systems. He suggests that the focus of narrowly targeted programmes can sometimes seem at least to benefit the agency rather than the original issue. He concludes:

> Give them more money, the cancer charities claim, and they will find the magic formula that will save us all from a hideous death. But could it be possible that that we are dying so that they might live?
> Monbiot (2001), p23

It is very healthy for agencies and also health systems to ask whether they have become ends in themselves or are still means to an end and, if so, what *is* that end?

The 'wonder drug' antibiotic has done much to bolster our culture's quasi-magical belief in dramatic, interventionist medicine although there has been over recent years a growing awareness of the dangers of antibiotics. Drug resistance is only one of the serious consequences of the abuse by health workers of the 'wonder drug'. The failure, however, to produce an equivalent drug to deal with viruses, whether those involved in the common cold or AIDS, has meant that medicine as magic has needed the boost that genetic medicine has brought to the picture. Once again, thanks to genetic medicine, we are led to believe that we can look to science and technology to produce the answer to the world's health problems – and of course, be ready to pay the price.

TOWARDS A FULLER, MORE CONTEXTUALIZED SENSE OF HEALTH?

The focus of health systems remains an individualized, decontextualized treatment, with an emphasis on technical intervention. Moreover, as we have said, the preoccupation of these health systems is on the *pathological*: what is wrong and broken and needs fixing. Our health systems, as Illich (1975) said all those years ago, are in fact *disease* systems. The media and the world of popular TV entertainment perpetuate the glamour and the drama of high-tech medicine which captures the headlines and resources in most health/illness systems. The focus, then, of these disease-oriented health systems is generally acute conditions, those involving 'muscular' interventions.

The thinking behind the National Health system in the UK at the time of its creation was that medicine and the hospital services should be, as Blane points out, 'part of a broader plan for social progress'; he goes on to remind us that the UK National Health Service was designed to deal with disease, but 'disease was only one of the "five sources of misery" which were to be eliminated by the reforms' (Blane et al, 1996). Unfortunately, the predictable happened and the health system became a system focused very much on disease in isolation from the other compounding sources of misery and, ultimately, ill health. Biomedicine, then as now, generally gets the lion's share.

It is interesting that even the good intentions of the visionaries of a comprehensive health system, as above, were still focused on *disease*, though at least in a more comprehensive, contextualized way, as one of the elements of 'misery' that had to be tackled by the state. This somewhat negative emphasis is understandable, given that the context was a Europe recently decimated by a horrendous war in which millions had been killed and maimed. *Health* was the intention, even if the immediate perspective was on the negative. The 21st century is also a century of war and disease, but even in this context we have to think outside of this framework and begin to think *health* and its maintenance, not just disease and its management.

In most countries, we have health systems that tend to decontextualize illness and health. Of course, faced with this as a bland statement, many health practitioners would deny the accusation: there have been moves to understand illness and health and well-being in their fuller human context, at least encompassing the psychological environment in which a patient lives. But, by and large, medical science remains a biological science of individual illness and not a science of human – individual and community – health.

There have been serious attempts to change this direction: it is to some of these significant steps towards a more balanced vision of health systems that the next chapter turns.

2

STEPPING AWAY FROM THE
MEDICAL MODEL: THE IMPORTANCE
OF CONTEXT

If you have come here to talk about brown bread and jogging, you can
... go away.

> Cathy McCormack, a committed Scottish health
> activist from Glasgow in Scotland, in the context
> of damp housing and ill health

This chapter traces the historical efforts, notably those inspired by
the World Health Organization, to move beyond the limitations
imposed by a narrow biomedical framework. A major part of this
can be seen as an attempt to include the idea of context or environment into the picture of disease and health.

PUBLIC HEALTH: THE IMPACT OF THE PHYSICAL
ENVIRONMENT

'Environment and health' in the mind of western-trained health personnel and many populations is an area taken care of by 'public
health' departments. These have a very honourable heritage in the
tradition of such people as John Snow, the man who, famously, by
linking cases of cholera in London to the source of drinking water,
laid the foundations of environmental health (Snow, 1855) and the
'tool' of public health, epidemiology. Virchow also has his claim to
fame here:

> *If medicine is to fulfil her great task, then she must enter the political*
> *and social life. Do we not always find the diseases of the populace*
> *traceable to defects in society? If disease is an expression of individual*

life under unfavourable circumstances, then epidemics must be indica-
tive of mass disturbances.

Virchow (1859)

The success of the public health tradition has been on the grand scale, with general admission that the great public works of hygiene and housing and the supply of clean water sources in Europe have made a huge impact on efforts to improve health and to reduce disease. Unfortunately, since major changes have been made in the environment, like the safe disposal of human waste, environment issues have often been considered as having been 'taken care of' and become divorced from health systems.

If one is to adopt a less Euro-centric perspective, worthy of note in this regard are the ancient historical experiences of cities like Mohenjo Daro in pre-Christian civilizations of the Indus Basin (Pankhania, 1994) and many have been awestruck at the sight of the remains of similar public health civil engineering in the ruins of earlier cultures in such countries as Sri Lanka. In Europe, prior to the impact of the public sewage and water schemes, many cities showed a pattern of infectious diseases and high infant mortality similar to that of present day 'Third World' societies. I have pointed out elsewhere the unfortunate loss or drastic dilution of this dimension of western health systems in the model of health care that was exported to the Third World during the colonial period (Macdonald, 2000). When newly independent countries looked for a model of health care to follow, what they had inherited as part of their 'development' model was the distorted framework elaborated in Chapter 1, with an enormous emphasis on treatment and cure of disease at the expense of prevention and the promotion of health and healthy environments. In good faith these countries developed an almost totally decontextualized system of care, dealing with symptoms in isolation from the milieu in which the illness was nourished. Some might argue that this was inevitable, given the fact that colonizing powers by definition are outside a lot of that context, that milieu: the social, cultural and spiritual world of patients using western-type medical institutions that sought to replicate European systems inevitably lie outside the knowledge and sympathy base of this medical system. This imbalanced heritage persists into the 21st century, so that often what money there is in poorer societies goes into curative care with almost negligible amounts spent on the creation of healthy environments, and few attempts are made to incorporate the psychological, cultural and spiritual context of people into health systems. An added terrible irony for countries that are dependent on the west for technical medicine is the inequitable difference in costs between 'developed' and 'developing' countries of life-enhancing pharmaceutical products. As one commentator says about a particular product which prevents mother-to-child transmission of HIV:

> *[it] costs $430 per 100 units in Norway, where there is hardly any market for it, she said, and $874 in Kenya, where the need is desperate. Drug prices in Norway are about average for European Union prices, which are generally lower than American ones.*
>
> McNeil (2000)

This is not to ignore the excellent work done in developing countries by many people who struggle to create healthy environments for their populations. The intention here is simply to highlight that the overwhelming impact of the globalization of western medicine is to have created an enormous emphasis on technical 'solutions' and, in particular, on pharmaceuticals and clinical interventions, thereby draining money away from primary health and preventative work and the creation of healthy environments.

FROM CONTEXT TO INDIVIDUAL BEHAVIOUR

Moreover, in the west itself, public health specialists, lacking great epidemics to monitor and seeing their domain increasingly privatized, are not always very clear as to the role of public health, and the task assigned to these workers is often little more than to police, with greater or lesser authority and therefore effectiveness, the negative impact on the environment of industry and such phenomena as vehicle pollution. Sometimes, given the individualizing tendency of 'health' services, some 'public health' programmes are involved in anti-smoking 'health promotion' campaigns which emphasise the importance of individual behaviour change, again in isolation from

the context of this behaviour. The landmark study of Hilary
Vaughan into reasons *why* people smoke seems to relegate context
into the too hard basket. Her study showed that a large part of the
explanation, the reason, for 'risky individual health behaviour' in the
group she examined was that smoking in working-class English
women smokers lay in their context – often of poverty and isolation
(Graham, 1986). Such insights necessitate adding a dimension of
complexity to over-simplistic attempts to effect behavioural change
and, in this case, to acknowledge smoking as an understandable coping strategy. The enormous reduction in smoking habits in the west
(in Australia, there has been a largely uninterrupted decline in smoking prevalence since the early 1960s, when an estimated 58 per cent
of men and 28 per cent of women smoked, compared with 19.5 per
cent of people over 14 years of age in 2001 (Chapman, 2003)) owes
a lot more to the political and social actions that attacked the companies profiting from this habit than to any 'don't do this' campaigns,
often offensive in their reductionism and refusal to see smoking 'in
context'. The flight of many tobacco companies to Third World
countries with their enormous advertising campaigns associating
smoking with western sophistication verges on the obscene. There
will be an inevitable increase in the use of hospital services in these
countries by those suffering from the effects of this 'sophistication'.
Double globalization: export the problem and export the 'solution'.

Historians might wonder why, after such great success and enormous evidence of the need to see environment as part of health systems, this perspective of health-as-environment has remained
largely confined to departments of public health, by and large her-
metically sealed from 'medicine' and acute care, as well as from
debates about rational allocation of the health dollar. The division
has meant that public health is generally seen as the poor cousin of
clinical care. Some departments of public health, conscious of this
lesser status and often led by doctors, sometimes rename themselves departments of 'Public Health Medicine', presumably to
remind the world that they are still part of the magic medical cir-
cle. Be that as it may, the bulk of the health dollar still goes to the
hospital and acute medicine. Sewers are hardly glamorous: it is
hard to envisage a TV programme in which the heroes and hero-
ines are civil engineers specializing in the safe disposal of human
waste competing for prime viewing time with those numerous

glossy shows which show handsome heroes bravely combating ill-ness with stethoscopes – or much more complicated technology – in state-of-the-art hospitals. It seems there will always be place for the series on doctors in Accident and Emergency services, espe-cially with helicopter back-up.

As we have said, western health systems are certainly not orga-nized in such a way that encourages public health and clinical health 'wings' of the system to function together as a whole. Somehow, the environment, seen as the physical environment, is conceived as being 'out there', having some connections with health but not con-ceptually or operationally to be considered in terms of planning. There is a wonderful story that a European health authority had dedicated monies to improve housing on the basis that poor hous-ing was the cause of many of the symptoms of respiratory infections which they were dealing with. Although the story turned out not to be true, no one could deny the rationality of the approach: spend money 'upstream', prevent the illness from happening in the first place and save money on unnecessary hospitalization.

'COMMUNITY HEALTH'?

What, then, is 'community health'? The words have less interna-tional currency than 'public health', although in the American tradition, 'community health' is still a respectable profession for doctors and nurses and refers to generally curative activities out-side the confines of the hospital, though often linked to it (De Voe, 2003). Elsewhere, the intention of community health advocates to create 'hospitals without walls' is seen as an honourable goal, with the focus squarely on the treatment of illness, though perhaps nearer to where the patient lives and therefore excluding from the planning equation the cost of hospitalization. Some versions of community health, as in the Australian context, represent genuine attempts to bring preventive and treatment work closer to the community. In the 1970s the political will seemed there to make this a reality (Rainbow Books, 1977). What is left of community health in Australia is an often underfunded, diluted version of this ideal with the focus on Mother and Child services and some other work for community nurses. By and large, doctors, and the inevitable health dollar which is associated with them, have little involvement with 'community health' and large sectors of the community do not see it as having relevance for them.

Left to itself (i.e. without considerable pressure from an informed public and a political vision), medicine in most countries tends to continue largely unchallenged down the technical, individualized road of the 'medical model'. Historians of the health care system in the UK will surely note the impact of the Thatcher vision of society: 'There is no such thing as society, only individuals' was one of the slogans of this most conservative of political leaders. This drastic myopia serves to shore up a doctor-centred, high-tech view of health, conveniently ignoring the wider social and economic contexts of health, conflates this with *health (i.e. disease) care* and allows the erosion of any political commitment to issues such as equity and community development for health. The simple logic of the proposition that 'improving the health of the whole population and the conditions for health in society is improving the health of the individuals in it' seems to have got lost. The emphasis on the supremacy of the *individual* in what we can call the 'anti-socialist approach' suggests that the well-being of the group is pursued mainly through the aggregated well-being of individuals.

PRIMARY HEALTH CARE AND HEALTH AS ENVIRONMENT

The 1960s and 1970s witnessed an international movement that was based on 'another development' (see, for example, the series *Development Dialogue*, 1972; and WHO, 2004a). In the view of some commentators on social development in the developing countries there was a perception that 'modernization' on its own, in terms of copying western technical development, an approach espoused by 'aid' to developing countries and many of the leaders of these countries themselves, was not delivering improved quality of life for the majority of people. This discontent with received wisdom about development in general was echoed by some in the health world by a realization of the failure of the dominant medical model to meet the major health needs of many countries and populations. This was particularly noticeable when, as was usually the case, clinical care became cut off from any real connection with public health. Although clinical care and departments of public health did not always work hand in hand in 'developed' countries, in many cases the hospital infrastructure was built on a civil culture that took for granted the great achievements of the public health era, at least in terms of clean water and the safe disposal of human waste. No such foundation existed in 'developing' countries: their health systems were based on European-type hospital systems. As we have said, this was a truncated and fatally flawed model of a health system, destined to serve badly the newly emerging nations that copied it. It could treat disease (*some* of the disease experienced by *some* of the population) but it couldn't build health. Lesley Doyal (1979) has articulated well the disruptive impact of colonialism on the health of colonized people. In most of these countries, the entire social, cultural, political and economic balance underwent cataclysmic change during the process of colonization. The provision of hospitals for African mine workers living hundreds of miles from their original communities may seem like a health positive. But in fact this practice was merely ensuring a productive workforce largely for the benefits of a white minority while the whole basis for health of entire communities and the individuals in them had been disrupted, politically, spiritually, economically and culturally. In such cases it is not just that western medicine 'decontextualizes': the patients in such hospitals were totally decontextualized, as were their families.

Another development, another health system

It was the very starkness of this misfit, these very contradictions, which gave rise to questioning. Another way of seeing health and doing health care began to emerge, with attempts to articulate another way of envisioning health and health care than the one underpinning the globalized version of health care that was coming from the west. The failure of the model was particularly poignant and apparent in so-called developing countries. Many of these had made considerable investments in that model, constructing a medical system based largely on hospitals and the deployment of western-trained personnel. But health problems persisted: low life expectancy and high infant mortality were the norm rather than the exception. Despite considerable expenditure in western-type health care, these problems persisted. There was a clear *prise de conscience* of this situation at the World Health Assembly of the WHO in 1977. The Director General of the WHO at the time, Hafden Mahler, had a keen sense of the problem and of the need for a new vision. The slogan that emerged as part of the attempt to promote change was 'Health for All', drawing attention to one of the basic criticisms of the gaps in health care services: lack of equity. These systems were especially deficient in addressing the needs of poorer people. A major theme that surfaced was the need for health care systems to put more emphasis on prevention of disease as opposed to the then almost exclusive concentration of effort on treatment and cure and institution-based systems of care. A WHO/UNICEF international conference was held in the former Soviet Union to promote the development of a movement to build another approach to health care policy. The movement was called Primary Health Care (PHC) (Macdonald, 2000) and the name of the town where the conference took place has become associated with the ideas of the movement: Alma Ata.

Primary Health Care and environment

PHC can be seen as representing a genuine movement *away* from systems of health care that perpetuate the separation between the curative and preventive wings of health care and begins, however tentatively, to articulate the need to acknowledge *context* as an essential element in any equation concerning health. In the document of the conference that launched the movement, there is an understanding of health systems which calls for their re-orientation and, at least implicitly, for a greater acknowledgement of the impact of the context of people's lives on their well-being. Underlying the document there is a recognition of the importance of *health* and not just *disease* and there is an understanding that health is determined (even if this word is not used) by such factors as education, inequalities in society, as well as cultural and other social factors. Medical historians should see the Declaration of the Alma Ata conference as among the first global expressions of the need to integrate a vision

of the environment and the social context of health into our understanding of health and health care planning.

As we look back from the vantage point of the new century,
Alma Ata and the Declaration of Primary Health Care represent an
idealistic aspiration for a more participatory, more just and more
interdisciplinary approach to health systems. What have been
called the 'three pillars' of PHC: participation, equity and intersectoral collaboration (Tarimo and Creese, 1990; Macdonald,
2000), help provide a vision of a health system which combines the
two classical wings of health systems, the treatment and the preventive, in the same conceptual and operational framework. It
seems that this vision was to a large extent the brainchild of Hafden
Mahler, the then Director General of the WHO. Historically, it
certainly represented in international terms an attempt to move
away from policies and planning related to health care systems
which place most of the emphasis and resources on *disease* managed
by institutional-based care and treatment and the modern technologies that accompany these. There is a clear acknowledgement
of the role of prevention, and the building of sustainable health in
the community, in the context of people's lives, where health is
either fostered or eroded. Though the word 'context' is not used in
the texts of the conference, it is clear that the philosophy of
Primary Health Care is built on a broad holistic view of health
which takes for granted the importance of the context of health and
how this context can be either enhancing or impeding.

Acknowledging equity is acknowledging context

A slogan was Health for All, drawing attention to one of the basic
criticisms of the gaps in health care services: inequity seems inbuilt.
Health services tend to be especially deficient in addressing the
needs of poorer people. In the fourth quarter of the 20th century
health technologies could be seen as having advanced dramatically,
but so had the gap in health status, as Alma Ata put it, between
countries and between groups within countries. From the beginning there was a moral tone about the document that launched
Primary Health Care. Health for All as a slogan draws attention to
the fact that this (health for all) is what we should be aiming for but

do not yet have. Depending on one's point of view, this is either a firm foundation for a debate on health care systems and policies related to them or it is simply either a pious exhortation or an indication of the philosophical rather than the pragmatic base of the Primary Health Care debate. That the moral dimension of the health system should be drawn into the discussion is surely a positive thing. In clinical training, whether of doctors or nurses or other health professionals, the discussion of ethical considerations often gets conveniently limited to the duty of care of individuals, micro-ethics as opposed to macro-ethics.

THE MORAL DIMENSION AND PROFIT

There is a tension in this dynamic which, in my opinion, receives insufficient attention at the level of the implementation of health care systems. On the one hand, there is the discourse of health care as a *vocation*, a noble calling which is embedded in a tradition of patient-centredness with the emphasis on service rather than personal gain (this discourse is implicit in the Hippocratic Oath and the nurse training which pursues the noble ideals of Florence Nightingale). On the other hand, there is a discourse that has its origins in the tradition of health care as an *economic business* like any other, one of the services which one purchases in a manner that corresponds to one's economic and social status. We can speak of the 'commodification' of health care: the same processes which bring about changes in the make and model of the car one drives affect the quality and cost of the health care one purchases.

This moral tone was part of the backdrop to the emergence of the Health for All policy of the WHO, both in the documentation around Primary Health Care and the programmes that followed it, like the Health Promotion movement. The introduction by the WHO of the notion of equity in the Health for All movement and its inherent principle, of access to health care as a *right*, has had the effect of obliging most national health policies to address the issue. Some would say that this has produced only a rhetoric, but for others it has proved a vehicle for change.

Alma Ata not only denounced the unacceptable nature of inequalities in health services between and within nations, it denounced inequalities in health status. Most people would acknowledge the links between poverty and ill health and that the improvement in the standard of living of any given population will impact on their health status. The call for equity in health is therefore often seen, rightly, as a political statement and the political nature of any given government will influence how this call is addressed in those circumstances.

A major theme that surfaced during this *prise de conscience* was the need for health care systems to put more emphasis on *prevention* of disease as opposed to then almost exclusive concentration of effort on treatment and cure and institution-based systems of care. This represents an acknowledgement of the need to manipulate the context of people's lives, of course with their consent, either to foster health or curtail illness. In response to the criticisms concerning the *disease* orientation of 'health' systems, there was a growing awareness of the need to promote conditions which foster *health*. This, of course, is in line with the well-known definition of health put forward by the WHO:

> *Health is not merely the absence of disease but the total physical, psychological and social well-being of individuals and communities.*

Primary Health Care is seen by some as a weak and ineffectual rhetoric, a smokescreen for the refusal to address the real issues of income distribution which cause ill health (Navarro, 1986). More sympathetic historians of health care may perhaps see it as an expression of a global search for rational and humane health systems; rational and humane, since Primary Health Care calls for the human to be at the centre of health systems' thinking and action – as *human*, not just as recipient of medicine. None of this contradicts the fundamental assertion of critiques like those of Navarro: improve the living condition, context, of people's lives and by and large their health will improve. The call for equity is a call for social change, for justice, a rejection of situations where people are not allowed the basic means of decent survival.

WHAT'S IN A NAME?

There are many people who strive for a better system, more balanced, more humane and more rational, and don't call it 'Primary Health Care'; many of these would even dismiss the name out of hand. Given the dominance of the focus on cure and treatment and the neglect of funding everywhere for prevention and promotion of health, it is clear that there would be enormous advantage in having a vocabulary that is shared by those who struggle at the prevention end of the spectrum for a more balanced system, a more rational mix of prevention and treatment, and who see the importance of people's environment on their health. Primary Health Care was an attempt to offer us such a vocabulary. By the first decade of the 21st century the language of Primary Health Care was still a matter of dispute to some and of indifference to others. Primary Health Care in the UK, without a strong tradition of community health other than such relative small programmes such as the admirable tradition of health (nurse) visitors, is generally taken to mean the work of general practitioners and 'progress' measured in the building up of hospital services in GP practices. As Walton pointed out years ago, even a few years after the launch of Primary Health Care at Alma Ata, most doctors in the UK or in Europe had never heard of the WHO's initiatives in this regard (Walton, 1983, 1985). There is still a need to find a common language; otherwise how can we talk of shared ideals, how can we challenge the imbalance and the contradictions, how can we be united with others who work in similar ways, who seek in different environments to build more rational and humane systems through training, education and resource allocation?

'Primary' as in 'primary school' or just as 'first contact'?

Primary Health Care as a concept tried, in however imperfect a way, to hold together the two wings of the health care system. It called for a system of treatment based on the basic or primary needs of particular communities. This is the (probable) meaning of the word 'primary' in Primary Health Care. It has often been misunderstood and taken to mean only the first line of contact between a given population and a health care delivery system, the medical system. As presented by Alma Ata, a Primary Health Care system *does* mean the first line of contact between need and medical provision but not *only* that. The focus of the entire health system should be on the primary needs of the community in question: a system of health care turned towards the needs of that community. The system is called upon to deal with the presenting symptoms – the *problem* – but to address the causality behind this problem as well. The logic of this is inescapable: if the common or *primary* complaints of a community are related to the communicable diseases of childhood, then the health care system, a Primary Health Care system, would focus on these conditions and, of course, aim to treat them as near to the community as possible. Secondary and tertiary care would support this focus, both by referral and by back-up. In the situation described, of communicable childhood diseases, these should not be usually dealt with at the level of hospital. Hospitals are not appropriate places to deal with diarrhoea, measles, acute respiratory infections and the like. In a Primary Health Care system these conditions would be dealt with as near to the community as possible.

Alternative names have been offered. It is said, with some justification, that Primary Health Care gets too easily subverted into primary *medical* care. In three different countries, general practitioners have looked assertively at me and declared: 'Primary Health Care? – we are Primary Health Care' and been none too pleased when I suggested they were indeed an important *part* of Primary Health Care rather than the whole phenomenon. Local vocabularies have sprung up to express the ideals of contextualized care, engaging with the environment and adding access to appropriate and affordable health care.

More important than names are the characteristics of the approach: the 'pillars' of PHC.

THE THREE PILLARS OF PRIMARY HEALTH CARE

Three of the main characteristics of the approach outline by PHC have been called its 'pillars': participation, equity and intersectoral collaboration (Macdonald, 2000). The Alma Ata conference called for *participation* of populations in decision-making about health, moving towards a model of interaction between people and professionals which challenges the notion of the patient and community as passive recipients. With its call for *equity*, it also took a moral stance: people have a right to health care and inequalities in health and health status are unacceptable. It further called for *intersectoral collaboration*, thereby adopting an understanding of health as being something created in the social domain, a precursor in this way of the *social determinant of health* literature. The conference highlighted the importance of other sectors in building the health of populations. The simple acknowledgement of the role of education and housing in the building and maintenance of health, to name only two of the relevant sectors that contribute to health, could have important consequences for the way we think and 'do' health in almost any country.

The Primary Health Care movement's insistence on the importance of the contexts of people's lives on their health must be seen as a manifestation of the growing appreciation of the social, economic and cultural underpinning of both health and disease. In the second half of the 20th century it was becoming increasingly difficult to ignore the insights coming from such disciplines as anthropology, political economy and sociology. All of these contribute to our understanding of the influences on health and disease to be found in the social world. Any attempts to reduce health to a decontextualized phenomenon and health care to a context-free technical operation become increasingly untenable, even irrational options. One explicit attempt to include the perspective of context in health is to be found in the Health Promotion movement.

A VISION OF A SYSTEM OF HEALTH CARE FOCUSING ON PEOPLE IN THEIR CONTEXTS

Primary Health Care, then, means a system of medical care and promotion of health focused on the health needs of a given community, in its particular circumstances or contexts, focusing on prevention and easy access to affordable care: a *whole* care system. We can think of populations dealing with poverty with infectious diseases of childhood with a system aiming at prevention, the creation of healthy environments but with access to the appropriate levels of health care when necessary. But what about a community where the disease pattern was different from that of a developing country with its high infant mortality and low life expectancy? What place for Primary Health Care in a 'typical' western community where the communicable diseases of childhood had largely been dealt with and the demographic shift was taking place so that the epidemiological pattern was of an ageing population with the chronic conditions of ill-health which one associates with this population? The same logic of a Primary Health Care system must still surely apply: a whole care system focused on the needs of that community with the emphasis on the primary needs of this ageing population. Again, secondary and tertiary care would be used appropriately, as referral and back-up. Hospitals would be used for acute cases that could not be dealt with at the community level. They should not be filled with older patients with chronic conditions who could be cared for in less medicalized situations and closer to and sometimes in their own homes. At its best, the notion of *early intervention* – dealing with problems before they become acute – makes perfect sense, not only for childhood conditions, but also at the other end of life's spectrum. We know that timely support for older people can stave off health problems and the need for hospitalization (WHO, 2002a).

In both scenarios (of childhood diseases and of ageing conditions of ill health), hospitals and their resources would be used more appropriately for those conditions which cannot be dealt with at the level of the community.

The shrinking hospital – An ambiguous concept

In its original conception, a successful integrated Primary Health Care system would mean an expanded community-based system of health care with access to an acute care system where appropriate. This is in fact the pattern that is predicted for the future of western-type medical systems. If we take the example of the British situation:

> *Across the NHS and Social Services in England, over 50,000 members of the allied health professions are providing patient centred care, working alongside doctors, nurses and scientists. They provide*

treatment and care across the range of health and social services, pro-
moting good health, treating patients who are acutely ill and caring
for those with chronic illnesses.

However, the role of the allied health professionals has too often been
undervalued or neglected. The Government is committed to chang-
ing this ... And we are committed to expanding the roles which the
allied health professionals play in health and social care.

NHS (2000), p5

The fact that this pattern – expanded community care, shrinking
hospitals – may come about for financial reasons should not be a
matter of surprise: the spiralling costs of acute care may likely
become the major driving force behind a move towards a more
rational balance between prevention and treatment and between
institutional and community-based care. Unfortunately, there is
cause for serious concern about this move towards shrinking the
hospital. Too often it does not indicate a genuine rebalancing of
resources between institution and community. Rather it is a cost-
cutting exercise: early discharge does not necessarily mean more
community support.

The types of services, needed away from the hospital setting, have not
received the planning, political and financial attention, to anywhere
near the same degree, that getting into, and receiving hospital ser-
vices, have in the past.

Community based nursing services and personal care services need to
be made more robust to be able to support these fundamental changes
across the NSW health system.

Council of Social Services NSW (2000)

There are moral and logical arguments in favour of a more balanced approach but to shift patterns of resource allocation in the
medical system from acute to community care requires more than
some advocacy for change from some high moral ground and a
shift of funds. Change in resource allocation in medical systems
does not happen easily. Often only the economic imperative can
alter well-entrenched patterns. Left to itself, institution-based

care, with its focus on treatment, becomes exorbitantly expensive and it is more likely to be economic managers in any setting who will rein in medical expansion and push for initiatives that keep people healthier and therefore out of hospital.

The logic of the Alma Ata arguments in favour of a Primary Health Care system as we have described is still compelling. The idea of a health care system keeping the balance between treatment and prevention and keeping an openness both to individual responsibility and government (at any level) obligation is surely a rational ideal. It means a re-thinking and re-planning of health care systems to keep this balance. The arguments in its favour apply in any society.

WHY IS THERE RESISTANCE IN THE WEST TO THE PRINCIPLES OF PHC?

Why, then, has Primary Health Care never or not yet been accepted in western societies? (It should be made clear that many individuals and groups embrace the philosophy of Primary Health Care: what has been lacking is not just the non-acceptance of the term in the west, but the use of Primary Health Care principles as the basis for planning for entire health systems.) Even where the logic of the arguments for a better balance has been acknowledged and policy statements been made in support of Primary Health Care, understood in the comprehensive way laid down at Alma Ata, the reality is often of a dual way of thinking and acting: a continuation of the division between treatment and prevention/promotion which has been the hallmark of western health care in the 20th century. This is despite some, even frequent, tokenistic acknowledgement of the need for community care and prevention.

I was present at the national planning of a Primary Health Care programme in an African country. The input into the discussion came from a variety of players, politicians, health department workers and health professionals with advice from international agencies. It became clear that a Primary Health Care system would involve a more rational distribution of resources between prevention and treatment, between town and country, between treatment and the building of healthy environments. At this point, a senior doctor took the floor and angrily demanded if this would involve turning funds away from hospital to the community. The response of the Minister of Health was telling and I think sounded the knell of any attempt to break the stranglehold of resources by curative care. 'Of course not, doctor', he said: 'we will continue with health care as we know it and the international agencies will help us with Primary Health Care'. They did, for a while. And what limited resources the government had went largely into curative care.

AN EXAMPLE FROM AUSTRALIA

The Public Health Association of Australia in its 1992 conference endorsed the principles of Primary Health Care:

> *Four key principles of the primary health care policy model are:*
>
> - *collaborative local networking (across all primary health care services, local government, consumers and community groups);*
> - *a more prominent role for the PHC sector in defining community needs and shaping paradigms of excellence;*
> - *support for informed and organised consumer and community involvement in health care decisions; and*
> - *a balancing of health care priorities between meeting micro and immediate needs on one hand and the macro and longer term issues on the other (addressing the former but in ways that also contribute to resolving the latter).*
>
> Public Health Association of Australia (2004)

This seems to have made no impact on the thinking or practice of the medical profession in the country for whom primary health care still means primary *medical* care. Part of the explanation for this misconception must lie in the education of health professionals, by and large focusing on the understanding and treatment of pathologies in individuals and, as has been said all along, decontextualizing these conditions.

There is, implicitly, in the Primary Health Care vision, a critique of western health care systems. The critique suggests that, *left to itself*, a typical western-type health care system can easily develop along lines that might mean the improvement of different aspects of medical technology and even medical practice, without necessarily involving the improvement of health status of communities (except of course through the tackling of disease if it presents itself) or even having this as its major preoccupation. Specifically, the mindset inculcated by such a health system allows the perpetuation of the draining of funds into technical medicine to the neglect of the creation of healthy environments. The separation means the perpetuation of the dominance of the 'downstream' approach. Of course, this sort of remark seems offensive to many hard-working health workers but, unfortunately, this is often a defensive reaction reflecting the old saying that a fish is often unaware of the water it swims in.

There have been several important conferences following Alma Ata, many extending the vision of what makes for health. Not least of these was the Rio conference, which set out some principles for the creation of a healthy global environment. The road from Alma Ata to Rio has made more explicit with each conference the importance of the environment in health. What is lacking has been a vision of health and health systems that helps us combine the quest for healthier environments as generally understood with the quest for more appropriate health care.

HEALTH PROMOTION

Alma Ata paved the way for the Ottawa Charter on Health Promotion in 1986 (Ottawa Charter, 1986), which spelled out the need to promote healthy environments and healthy social policies. This led to the notion of 'settings': the idea that health should be addressed in the context, the environment in which people live out their lives, whether their homes, their communities, schools or workplaces.

In this spirit, WHO initiatives like the Healthy Cities programme have offered frameworks to plan and execute integrated health systems that acknowledge the role of other sectors such as transport, schools and housing in the maintenance of people's health. Though the words used in such programmes may vary, what is being offered in such initiatives as these is the opportunity to plan environments which foster health in communities and the individuals in them. One of the aims of the Ottawa Charter was the 're-orientation of the health services'. Unfortunately, many committees set up to implement Healthy Cities programmes often lack the authority to command the attendance and participation of the power holders in the medical system, and so the imbalance between prevention and treatment persists. Without a mechanism with the brief to bring acute care to account and be part of a rational planning process for the health of communities rather than the management of disease and injury, Health Promotion has been labouring at its task of prevention.

Both Alma Ata and the Ottawa Charter represent, implicitly, a critique of the medical model. Unfortunately, nowhere in the world has either of them effected a significant global change in the model. Alma Ata, if known at all in the west, was considered fine for 'over there', meaning in a somewhat colonialist and therefore racist perspective, the so-called 'developing' countries. Health Promotion has been accepted in western industrialized countries as an optional 'cousin' of the health services, rather than an essential partner, often seen as a health education service and never as really threatening to overturn the preponderance of the clinical medical focus in terms of resource allocation and planning. Certainly no one would claim that it has in any significant way effected a 're-orientation of the health services'.

Foundations not built upon

The basic tenets of Health Promotion seek to enshrine the notion of the importance of context for health and its maintenance. The principles of Health Promotion, as outlined in the Ottawa Declaration of 1986, demonstrate this:

> *To reach a state of complete physical, mental and social well-being, an individual or group must be able to identify and to realize aspirations, to satisfy needs, and to change or cope with the environment. Health is, therefore, seen as a resource for everyday life, not the objective of living. Health is a positive concept emphasizing social and personal resources, as well as physical capacities.*

Therefore, health promotion is not just the responsibility of the health sector, but goes beyond healthy life-styles to well being.
                                                           Ottawa Charter (1986)

If these principles were genuinely valued, given status, built on and developed by all health services, medical schools and other training establishments like colleges of nursing, it would be relatively easy for all health workers to adopt an *environmental* notion of health: health services would be seen to be an essential *part* – but only a part – of the work of health services. Unfortunately, this is not the case and Health Promotion is conceived of, often by health promotion workers themselves, as an addition to health services rather than the agent of their re-orientation. Nevertheless, the Ottawa Charter can be seen as an historical landmark in international health policy in its endorsement of the central importance of the environment, however tentatively this is expressed.

Alma Ata and PHC were subjected to both *strong* and *weak* interpretations (Walsh and Warren, 1979; Wisner, 1988), the first version (strong) implying genuine change of health systems based on the three 'pillars', the second version (weak) involving no real change in the status quo but consisting of some 'add-ons' at the periphery of decision-making and policy (Macdonald, 2000). The same fate awaited Health Promotion: for some, there has always been a 'strong' version which seeks a new health system with re-oriented health care and a concerted movement towards policies and practices that create healthy environments, often with an emphasis on equity. For many others, however, Health Promotion has become simply another name for health education and delivering information about health and 'healthy lifestyles'. In the emphasis on lifestyles, the focus is on personal responsibility for improved health status and away from the political and social context of such lifestyles, a classical 'decontextualization' strategy of the medical model (Macdonald, 2000).

The task and challenge of a more comprehensive model remain, worldwide. There is still a chasm between the two wings of health care systems and there is still a great emphasis on the individual, both as the consumer of health care and as the person 'responsible' for their own health. Given the privatization of both curative and preventive measures and their consequent division into different 'companies', there is an even more urgent need for a vision of more rounded and balanced health systems which combine care and treatment with the promotion and maintenance of health in individuals and communities. The international conferences that followed Ottawa, notably the Rio Summit in 1992, continued the concern for healthy environments. Agenda 21 represents a huge milestone in our understanding of the need to create a global movement for healthy environments. Sadly, even the ecology movement's impact on the global health debate has not been to try to integrate existing processes of health promotion such as Healthy Cities. The praiseworthy calls for a sustainable environment do not seem to see earlier initiatives such as Alma Ata and the Ottawa Charter as worthy of attention. It is imperative to begin a synthesis: to see environmental concerns, health promotion concerns and health care concerns as being linked. Again, this implies is a call for humility – there is a sense in which the ecology movement seems to have captured the high moral ground in the development debate. There is a need to incorporate the messy, real world of health care into planning for healthy environments. To suggest that a healthy environment does not need to include access to appropriate and affordable health services is simply arrogant and not a true 'ecological' approach to health and health care. Even if the links with the ideas behind PHC and Health Promotion and more recent ecological perspectives are not generally acknowledged by the 'green' movement, it is not hard to see a logical development between Ottawa and the Health Promotion Charter of 1986 and the Rio Summit of 1992. 'Sustainable Development' must begin to promote a vision of environments, global and local, which sustain health in its widest sense and not shun the necessary partnership with health services.

A NEW PARTNERSHIP

On the side of health services, as has been said, we need a system of health care that combines, conceptually and operationally, the imperatives of prevention and promotion on the one hand and treatment and cure on the other; but there needs also to be a reaching out to the insights provided by the ecology movement. Any conceptualization which allows them to be thought of as totally separate systems will, by the same token, allow the treatment side of the equation to continue to dominate not only the thinking and planning of health care systems but also their budgets. The perceptions and energies of the movement of Agenda 21 (Rio Declaration on Environment and Development, 1992) and for a healthy planet must find a way to include the personal, the emotional and the spiritual dimensions of people's environments, as well as the right of every individual to be part of an environment that offers them access to necessary health care.

Of course, since the concept of Primary Health Care means a framework balancing treatment with prevention and promotion, in a single system there would also be systems in place to attempt to *prevent* the primary conditions in the first place: in the case of communicable diseases of childhood, this would mean activities to promote the health of children and this would inevitably involve a health care system focused also on the environment and its improvement, the creation of health-promoting environments. Even though this vocabulary of *environments* does not feature in the text of Alma Ata, it is clear that the ideas are there. In the other context of a population of at least potentially chronically ill elderly people, often living in isolation, the same imperatives would apply: genuine efforts to provide care in the community and to provide environments that sustain the psychological and physical well-being of older people. Health workers are being asked, under the name of *intersectoral collaboration*, to work with all those sectors which contribute to health, including agriculture, education and housing. As we have seen, the Primary Health Care notion of health takes for granted the fact that schools, workplaces and homes all play a vital role in the sustaining of health (and these points were actively taken up, of course, as we have seen, by the Health Promotion movement).

MORE EVIDENCE OF THE NEED FOR A CHANGE IN PERSPECTIVE AND PRACTICE

Until relatively recently, the call for more emphasis on prevention and for a more equitable and rational balance in the distribution of the health dollar has been seen as a moral imperative. And indeed it is; there *should* be a better balance. But especially in the last few years there has arisen a body of scientific evidence that needs be drawn into the debate. The work on the 'social determinants of health' increasingly highlights the irrationality of an overemphasis on medical technical interventions to the neglect of the health-enhancing or health-threatening contexts in which people live out their lives. It is to this body of evidence we now turn in the next chapter.

3

THE SOCIAL DETERMINANTS
OF HEALTH

Even among the small proportion of modern causes of death where medical competence is greatest, mortality rates appear to be influenced more by environmental than by medical factors.

Mackenbach et al (1990)

THE CENTRAL ROLE OF CONTEXT IN THE HEALTH OF INDIVIDUALS AND COMMUNITIES

In the earlier chapters it has been argued that many of the policies and practices of our health systems continue to perpetuate reductionist views of how health is maintained; they pursue the analogy of bodies as machines which, if they break down, can be fixed by the use of ever more expensive and complicated medical technology (supplemented by some individual responsibility for personal behaviour). However, there have always been powerful arguments that would suggest that this partial view of the phenomenon of health creates a distortion of perception and practice. There have always been voices, in most cultures, which draw attention to the centrality of environment, *milieu*, context, to the notion of health. Among the most cogent of these more recent arguments in western society (we shall turn to other cultures later) are those to be found in the body of knowledge that we can describe as the 'social determinants of health' literature, providing striking fresh evidence of the fact that health and illness are linked, inextricably, to the social, cultural, economic and emotional environments of individuals and communities. Health is not just situated in the environment: it must be seen as the very interaction between the self/community and the environment.

It is striking that this evidence of the centrality of context is emerging despite the persistent, almost religious-like statements of confidence in the new wonderful techniques of biomedicine waiting for us just around the corner to usher in an era of achievable perfect health. The latest of these can be found in the promises of the new magic medicine of genetic science, as we have seen in an earlier chapter in the quote from Crenson:

> ... the new information [about the genome] is expected to revolutionise drug development, making it much easier for pharmaceutical companies to target their products at the actual causes of disease. (emphasis added)
>
> Crenson (2000)

The quote is worth repeating since it shows neatly the link between the continuing belief of allopathic thinking around targeting specific aetiology, one single cause, often biological, for an episode of illness, and the commercial concerns of interested parties, in this case the pharmaceutical companies specializing in medical technology which would offer the bullets to hit this target. Again, the complexity of human health and illness is simplistically reduced: even in today's world where the reality of co-morbidity (Australian Government, Department of Health and Ageing, 2004) and multiple aetiology (Focosi, 2001) is widely acknowledged, we are still being lured into hopes of a 'pill (or at least a genetic manipulation) for every ill'.

Providing a much-needed balance to this 'faith' or mindset, we have literature on the research into the social determinants of health which provides us with a very powerful strand of evidence reminding us that health is inextricably linked to context, to environment. Common sense tells us that health is at least closely linked to our surroundings – our physical, social and spiritual context – and that health has something to do with the interaction of human beings with this environment. The studies on the *social determinants of health* give substance to this common-sense view by providing us with empirical evidence of this impact.

The work on the social determinants of health has often emerged from considerations about differentials in health status: concerns as to why some people and groups of people have poorer health outcomes than others. At the same time there has been an increase in our collective knowledge of links between the body's physiology and the working of the mind. Often the brain mediates this link between the body and its environment either directly as the person encounters thoughts, ideas, non-material phenomena and reacts to these; or indirectly, as the mind interprets the physical phenomena it encounters – like cold, heat, smoke, physical deprivation like hunger, etc.

The evidence grows of the links between the social context and the individual's biological and mental condition, their health and well-being:

> *There is a chain that runs from the behaviour of cells and molecules to the health of populations, and back again, a chain in which the past and the present social environments of individuals and their perceptions of those environments constitute a key set of links. No one would pretend that the chain is fully understood, or is likely to be for a considerable period of time to come. But the research evidence currently available no longer permits anyone to deny its existence.*
>
> Evans et al (1994), p184

Context is more than just a contributory factor

It is under the banner of the social determinants of health that researchers have collected information about these 'key links' between social circumstances and the health of populations and, of course, of the individuals making up these populations. When we speak of the social determinants of health, we are looking at the factors in the social context of people's lives which contribute to and are an *essential dimension* of the creation and maintenance of health in individuals and communities.

THE NEED TO KEEP THE BIG PICTURE FIRMLY IN MIND

Some evidence has emerged that health services play only a minor role in maintaining the health of communities (Grzywacz and Fuqua, 2000). It is understandably hard for doctors and nurses and other professional health workers to acknowledge, not just intellectually, but in practice, that health care and health services have less of an impact on health than the circumstances of people's lives. With the globalization of western medicine it is fair to say that in most societies now the culture is so technology-focused that health systems and health expenditure are generally tied to medicine rather than to the context in which people live. Populations applaud the allocation of funds to research into treatment of asthma by the same authorities that do nothing to regulate the use of diesel fuel, known to be a major contributory factor in the causation of asthma. A further classic but tragic example of the gap between treatment and prevention is to be found in the situation of tobacco-related diseases. The first years of the 21st century witnessed the exposure of the inescapable negative impact of tobacco consumption on people's health: there is now no possible denial of the fact that cardiovascular disease, cancer, strokes and many other conditions are linked to smoking tobacco. Financial interest prevented this link from being recognized for many years. Now that the facts are in the open, the tobacco companies have turned their attention to the markets of the developing world. Many cities in these countries are festooned with advertisements promoting the idea that modernity is linked to smoking. What is absolutely certain is that in five years from now and ever after, there will be a growth in the 'health' industry: medicine and medical interventions will flourish dealing with the consequences of such preventable conditions: stroke, cardiovascular illness, cancers and surgical interventions, many of them highly complex and expensive like bypasses and heart transplants. The development of these 'health' initiatives, 'downstream', will be as a direct result of the encouragement of ill health 'upstream': an environment which facilitates cigarette smoking.

All this is a reminder that 'health is politics'. The 'microscopic' perspective, the narrow focus on biological malfunctioning and its rehabilitation, allows us not to focus on the 'macroscopic' vision (Macdonald, 2000) and pretend that health work is not political. However, it becomes increasingly difficult to argue that the big picture – the way, for example, that society's benefits are shared out – is not a major determinant of health, as we shall see. It is not only within countries that the health impact of political decisions is felt (the case of allowing multinationals to promote and sell tobacco without impunity is a case in point). The political economy between countries as, for example, in the terms of trade, has a huge impact on creating an environment which either fosters or hinders health. At the time of going to press, the Australian government and the newly independent East Timorese government are attempting to finalize shared maritime borders. Arguably, if Australia does get the larger share of the cake, as seems likely to be the case, East Timor will be denied the possibility of building an adequate infrastructure, including health service institutions which will lift the country out of poverty. Health *is* politics, sometimes macro, sometimes micro politics.

There are, of course, many social 'determinants' of health and they vary from location to location and between the circumstances of different groups. As we shall see, the very differences between groups, certainly as experienced by those doing less well, can themselves be seen as a determinant.

AND WHAT OF PERSONAL RESPONSIBILITY?

Not all 'causality', of course, lies in the social sphere. In addition to the genetic inheritance each person has, there is the matter of one's personal behaviour and attitude: most people have some agency in their reaction to the circumstances of their lives with consequent impact, for good or ill, on their health. In some understandings of health that underpin health systems the world over, the major determinants of health are often taken for granted as being situated in the triangle of genetics, health care and personal behaviour. Talk shows and popular literature buy into this vision of things. No one could deny that personal behaviour has an impact on health but this behaviour is often mediated through the social and economic circumstances of those who are 'behaving badly'. Adverse social circumstances might mean we are 'blaming the victim' and, as Jarvis and Wardle (2000, p241) put it, this approach is 'unhelpful, in that it fails to address underlying questions of why disadvantaged people are drawn to these behaviours and the nature of the social individual influences that maintain them'.

For me, one of the major reinforcing learning experiences of this truth was in an exchange with Cathy McCormack, a committed health activist from Glasgow. I had arrived to interview her for a Primary Health Care newsletter. Her organization had highlighted the role of damp housing in the ill health of families in Scotland. The large housing 'schemes' in Scotland are classic examples of contexts of multiple social disadvantage, where lack of opportunity for jobs, decent housing, transport and the like combine to provide a complex and sometimes devastating cocktail. Lack of facilities and damp housing were some of the predictable 'determinants of health' in her context. Her opening remark was that if I had come to talk of 'brown bread and jogging', I could get lost, or words to that effect. The value of the personal decisions and behavioural control involved in 'brown bread and jogging' are not in doubt, but we need to move towards an understanding of health and a practice of health care that enshrines the wisdom of people like Cathy McCormack, in which 'health' is inextricably linked to the context of people's lives. Personal behaviour and lifestyle will always be easy targets for reductionist approaches to 'health promotion', especially when there is vested interest in drawing attention away from those social determinants of health which lie in the socioeconomic disadvantage which many people in many countries experience. We need a contextualized understanding of health and a health service practice consistent with this vision. In many situations it is perfectly logical to say that health is environment, certainly as much environment as personal behaviour. And, of course, common sense should lead us to see that *health* lies in the dynamic between personal agency and the environment. This is the message of Chapter 5.

ENVIRONMENT IN THE GRAND TRADITION OF PUBLIC HEALTH

The focus, in traditional public health policy and practice, tends to be on the material environment. And of course, historically, the public health movement has made a huge impact on people's health status in many industrialized countries, with its emphasis on environment and health, understood largely as having to do with clean and affordable drinking water, the safe disposal of human waste and decent housing. Operationally, public health tends to be separated from the organization and practice of the treatment wing of the health system. This is especially true with the increasing trend to put the services involved into the private domain. This means not only clinical services, but also 'outsourcing' public health services, a formula endorsed by agencies like the World Bank (World Bank, 1993). Crude versions of this 'commodification' of services abound, services which had often been regarded as essential building blocks of health to be not only guaranteed by government, but carried out by government, whether local or regional. Access to water is often a good indicator of the 'health' of the public health system in any country:

> *Water is the essence of life. Without water human beings cannot live for more than a few days. It plays a vital role in nearly every function of the body, protecting the immune system – the body's natural defences – and helping remove waste matter.*
>
> *But to do this effectively, water must be accessible and safe. Lack of safe water is a cause of serious illnesses such as diarrhoeal diseases which kill over 2 million people every year (the vast majority children, mostly in developing countries). Contaminated water whether drunk or used to cook food, harms people's health. Water is also essential for hygiene, growing food, keeping animals, rest, exercise and relaxation and for a variety of social and cultural reasons.*
>
> WHO (2004b), p6

In the year 2000 I witnessed in the Bolivian city of Cochabamba a heartening (albeit temporary) dropping of social barriers between rich and poor in response to the privatization of water. Prices soared immediately to a ridiculous extent and people of all social classes took to the streets. The political response was rapid and the decision reversed (probably temporarily), while the forces of privatization withdrew to regroup and restrategize.

As privatization of the two wings of health services, curative and preventative, proceeds rapidly in our days, the chances of a system that will bind them together seem to recede with equal speed.

THE SOLID FACTS

The work on the social determinants of health has come as a timely reminder of the close link between our environment, understood in a very wide sense, and our biological, spiritual and mental health. As will be suggested, an expanded notion of environment can allow us to incorporate access to health services as an important part of the living 'environment' and give life to the notion of a genuine *health* system.

The WHO has popularized some of the research findings concerning the links between context and health in a remarkable and simple document called *Social Determinants of Health: The Solid Facts* (Wilkinson and Marmot, 2003). The determinants chosen for inclusion in this document by the WHO are:

1 the social gradient
2 stress
3 early life
4 social exclusion
5 work
6 unemployment
7 social support
8 addiction
9 food
10 transport.

Many of these factors have to do with the social fabric, the world with which people interact on a regular and constant basis. This expanding of the notion of environment is an essential step in the deepening of our understanding of the phenomenon that is health. Health lies squarely in the domain of this interaction.

We can turn to some of the social determinants highlighted by the WHO. They illustrate the importance of this expanded notion of environment for health and their straightforward text is backed up by references to important research in the area. These are 'solid facts', not just opinions.

Social gradient

Underlying much of the social determinants of health research is the growing evidence of the link between income and social status and the attendant literature that shows a concern for inequalities in society. We now have massive amounts of evidence of the common-sense position that being poor is bad for your health. Although, as we will see, the notion of relative well-being (how we fare in relation to others in terms of social advantage) is important, it is wholesome to acknowledge that our health depends, to a large extent, whether acknowledged or not, on the ability or otherwise to acquire the basic necessities of life for ourselves and those for whom we are responsible. Of course, these necessities vary in nature from society to society. As two of the important researchers say on this matter: the 'differences in morbidity and mortality between socioeconomic groups have been observed in many studies and constitute one of the most consistent findings in epidemiological research' (Lynch and Kaplan, 2000, p13). It is arguable that one of the reasons that there is not as much public debate about these issues as one would have expected, given the weight of the available evidence, is that this literature and the research embedded in it situates health and health care squarely in the political arena. The evidence thus provided gives the lie to the belief embedded in the justification for capitalist modernization expressed by Rockefeller a century ago and pursued relentlessly ever since: 'Misery is a technical problem' (Macdonald, 2000) and therefore susceptible to technical solutions. Resource allocation in health is generally skewed to feed the myth that the 'answer' to ill health lies in high-tech medicine, despite the accumulated evidence that the clustering and accumulation of psychosocial disadvantage is perhaps the most powerful determinant of health status. Addressing medical needs 'downstream' without addressing the 'upstream' conditions, in this case, of poverty, the inability to secure fundamental necessities to sustain a 'decent' life, must be one of the great contradictions of many modern societies.

The World Bank estimates that there are around 1.5 billion extremely poor people in the world. For those living in poverty the impact reaches far beyond income and monetary matters: the great-est adversities are the lost opportunities to develop essential human capabilities. Poverty is a disease that saps people's energy, dehuman-izes them and creates a sense of helplessness and loss of control over one's life. Illiteracy, ill health, malnourishment, environmental risks and lack of choices contribute to the perpetual cycle of poverty and ill health. Health is a vital asset for the poor. Without health, a person's potential to escape from poverty is weakened due to lost time, labour, income, and the burden of health care costs.

International Council of Nurses Fact Sheet (2004)

It is not simply lack of resources which impact on people's health, it is what people have to survive on in relationship to what others in their society have; this is part of what is meant by *social gradient*: where we are situated, relatively, on the ladder of prosperity. Some countries, like Canada, are increasingly acknowledging the impor-tance of addressing the gap between haves and have-nots as an essential preoccupation of effective health policies: 'Research shows that poor people are less healthy than rich people. Income distribution in a society is also a key element. The greater the gap between the richest and poorest people, the greater the differences in health' (Canada Health Network, 2004). It is not only that poverty is bad for your health, as common sense dictates; there is evidence that your position in social hierarchies affects your health. The fact is that, in general, the higher your status in the workplace and in society at large, the healthier you are likely to be and the longer you are likely to live in comparison with those further down the scale (Marmot, 1996). By the same token, those further up the scale are likely to live longer and enjoy better health. Of course, greater prosperity, in terms of material goods and access to money, does not guarantee better health, as the phenomenon of obesity and related conditions of ill health in 'affluent' societies testify.

There are differences in the way these 'facts' are understood. Most governments will shirk from drawing the conclusion that the best way to improve the 'health of the nation' is to improve the stan-dard of living of the whole population, for example, by ensuring a basic minimum wage, etc. This is despite the fact that the evidence points ever more closely to the *macroeconomic* context as a crucial 'determinant' of health. Individuals live out their lives impacted upon by economic factors often beyond their control:

> *We are just beginning to see the critical nature and function of extra individual factors such as institutions and communities as important agents in the socioeconomic stratification of the health of individuals and populations.*
>
> Lynch and Kaplan (2000), p30

The *Solid Facts* document of the WHO is clear on the policy implications of this acknowledgement of extra-individual factors:

> *Societies that enable all their citizens to play a full and useful role in the social, economic and cultural life of their society will be healthier than those where people face insecurity, exclusion and deprivation.*
>
> Wilkinson and Marmot (2003)

Those societies which refuse to take this perspective on board – of the basic link between health status and economic status – often embrace a more reductionist rhetoric of 'personal' responsibility, reinforcing the idea that health is principally an individual matter and, as has been said before, health gets decontextualized. Often this involves collusion between a narrow medical model and a conservative political agenda. The notion that 'health is the business of the individual' was mightily reinforced by such statements as Mrs Thatcher made when she was British Prime Minister: 'There is no such thing as society, only individuals'. The determinants of health literature gives the lie to this position. Building an environment that allows people the means of living decently is central to the health of any society and its individual members. An important part of *health* is the economic context in which a person lives out his/her life.

Education

In addition to socioeconomic status (and poverty) another obvious 'social determinant of health' is education; itself, of course, generally symbiotically linked to one's socioeconomic standing. The development literature (i.e. concerning 'Third World' countries) has been making the links between education, including literacy and health and ill health, for some years. But the reality is the same in all societies:

> *Statistics Canada reports that people with more than 12 years of education are less likely to have high blood pressure, high blood cholesterol, or to be overweight.*
> Saskatchewan Public Health Association (1999), p1

And in the European context, Blane and his co-authors tell the same story:

> *The most advantaged individuals in terms of education have the lowest mortality rates, and mortality rates tend to increase in a stepwise fashion as individuals become more educationally disadvantaged.*
> Blane et al (1996), p171

One can envisage education as that part of the environment which is set up to feed the minds and spirits of people, hopefully encouraging their self-confidence and their capacity to engage with 'the world' and, of course, in terms of training, equipping them to earn a living. The education one receives can either build up one's ability to engage 'successfully' with the environment or reinforce feelings of inadequacy or complacency at one's lot in life.

An image of health emerges as the 'successful' interaction between the self and the environment. The two mentioned determinants, social gradient and education, illustrate well the fact that the phenomenon of 'health' is often inextricably linked to the interaction between the individual and community and their context(s): a person's experienced position in life and their education either 'feed' or 'starve' their well-being and their ability to engage with other aspects of 'the world', like the domain of employment and social interaction. A child growing up with multiple choices in its life, the basic material needs well catered for, is in an environment which is health-enhancing; his/her mental and physical health is better placed to flourish than the child growing in a context of few choices and struggling to meet the requirements of his/her basic needs. Education intervenes: it either increases the child's self-confidence and purchasing power or else it doesn't, but either way it impacts on the child's interaction with its environment. Education is by definition in the business of assisting the person to deal well, and profitably, with the world in which they exist. Education therefore must be seen as a very important part of the environment capable of strengthening or undermining a person's engagement with their world.

Stress

We are constantly adding to our understanding of stress and its role in the maintenance or deterioration of health and it is often spoken of as a *determinant* of health. The WHO's excellent summary of the social determinants says that many psychosocial stresses can accumulate during the life course of any person and thereby increase the chances of poor mental health and even premature death. Social biology, the study of the impact of psychosocial factors on physical health, tells us that 'chronic stress, like acute stress, may lead to immunosuppression with possible increases in vulnerability to a range of diseases' (Brunner, 2000, p311).

> *In emergencies, the stress response activates a cascade of stress hormones that affect the cardiovascular and immune systems. Our hormones and nervous system prepare us to deal with an immediate physical threat by raising the heart rate, diverting blood to muscles and increasing anxiety and alertness. Nevertheless, turning on the biological stress response too often and for too long is likely to carry multiple costs to health. These include depression, increased susceptibility to infection, diabetes, and a harmful pattern of cholesterol and fats in the blood, high blood pressure and the attendant risks of heart attack and stroke.*
> Wilkinson and Marmot (2003), p8

It is in this context that *allostatic load* is spoken of. By this is meant the possibility of stress-induced damage to health. The great difference from some years ago in this regard is that it is no longer possible to dismiss physiological malfunctions which are stress related as being 'all in the mind' or purely 'psychosomatic', if by this we mean imagined symptoms. We are now much more able to begin to trace the complex links between mind and body and to chart the biological pathways in which stress impacts on the body. Brunner reminds us that dealing with stress is part of the normal functioning of human life. Problems arise, however, when stress is too much and the system is overloaded:

> *Frequent and prolonged activation of the flight-or-fight and other endocrine responses appear to be maladaptive ... and may prove to be central in understanding the social distribution of cardiovascular, infectious and other diseases.*
>
> Brunner (2000), p314

The immune system and psychoneuroimmunology

From what has already been said of what we could describe as the 'dance of health and illness', by which I mean the interaction between the person and his/her context, it has to be said that this context or environment plays a greater role than has generally been accepted in western medical-health thinking. Often the impact of the environment is mediated through the mind of the person involved. But it is important to note that this impact – of education, social gradient or social exclusion or inclusion – is, as has been said, not 'all in the mind'. Reference has already been made to the immune system. The issue of the immune system's response to the total environment and what has been called psychoneuroimmunology brings a new dimension to the arguments for a deeper understanding of this interactive 'dance of health and illness'. We are now accumulating evidence on the impact of the social environment on mental and *physical* health via very tangible effects on the body's immune system.

Work in this field since the 1980s by such researchers as Kiecolt-Glaser and colleagues has charted the impact – both negative and positive – on the immune system of social relationships, loneliness/sense of belonging, close relationships such as marriage (Kiecolt-Glaser et al, 1984, 1987; Glaser et al, 1985; Thomas et al, 1985; Cohen et al, 1997). It is not only that the subjects of the research *felt* less well when undergoing certain experiences (for example, loneliness); they were found to have lower levels of natural killer-cell activity during this experience. If the phenomenon of loneliness can have measurable impact on the body's ability to respond to disease, how much more impact must be involved in the ongoing stress of caring for a permanently disabled child or spouse or coping with major trauma such as war, occupation or bereavement?

Social inclusion and social support

So the environment, again, this time the emotional environment, is acknowledged as having an important impact on health. It is fundamental, in the real sense, to human health, to be cared for. Human well-being is nourished not only by food, but by supportive engagement with other people, by the knowledge and experience of being cared for and valued. If the already mentioned link between health and an adequate material economic base seems obvious, so might also the insistence in the same related literature about this matter of the importance for health of social support networks and social cohesion. The most memorable conference event for me over the last few years has been provided by Richard Wilkinson, an academic whose contribution in this field has also been very significant, concluding a conference on health promotion with his conviction, academically supported, that what adds years to life is belonging to a supportive social network on the one hand and the experience of being loved on the other (Wilkinson, 2000). This is quite striking in the face of the already mentioned tendency in health promotion to emphasize the role of the individual in maintaining his or her health by avoiding at-risk behaviour, but there was some wonderful irony in a social scientist of global stature telling health managers and workers that to reduce morbidity and add years to life, 'what you need is love' (although he may not have used these terms).

Berkman and Glass (2000) follow Kahn and Antonucci in defining social support as being 'transactional in nature involving both giving and receiving' (p145). More straightforwardly, perhaps, Cobb sees it as referring to the situation in which a person believes that he/she 'is cared for and loved, is esteemed and valued and belongs to a social network of communication and mutual obligation' (Cobb, 1975, p301). Such a perspective helps us enlarge our notion of 'environment': our health is sustained or threatened, nourished or diminished by not only our physical and economic environment and our interaction with it, but our emotional environment, our sense of belonging and being valued. Again, this seems like common sense; (nearly) every family knows it: your children and your partner need not only food and clothing but also someone supportive to come home to. Everybody does. That there are biological pathways in this link between social support and well-being is almost beyond dispute (Kubanski et al, 1998); the exact nature of these pathways is another matter. The tendency to focus on the pathological in 'health' services has meant that such studies as there have been have often looked at negative emotional states as predictors of poor health outcomes. But Kubanski and Kawachi draw attention to some studies looking at the salutogenic (even if they do not use that expression – see Chapter 5 for a discussion of salutogenesis). They report Fredrickson's theory of 'broaden and build':

> *With positive emotion experiences, individuals may develop physical skills that build strength, cognitive skills that enhance coping and social-affective skills that aid in building and strengthening relationships. Such resources are, in turn, hypothesised to promote health and well being.*

Kubanski et al (1998), p67

In the context of social support, a useful distinction is made between social integration and social capital. Both are beneficial for health. *Social integration* means the positive connections any individual has with others; these could be friends, families, close ties with groups such as churches, clubs, etc. *Social capital* refers to characteristics of the *collective* itself which can contribute to the well-being of the population. Durkheim famously studied this phenomenon in relation to suicide, which, as Kawachi and Berkman point out, is 'one of the most individualistic acts imaginable'. 'Durkheim succeeded in demonstrating that the population rate of suicide is, in fact, related to collective features of society' (Kawachi and Berkman, 2000, p174). There is something in the society itself, independent of particular individuals, which either facilitates the route towards suicide, or, conversely, helps sustain people in life.

The research on these matters is of tremendous importance in enlarging our understanding of health and the central significance of context and our personal and collective interaction with this context.

Drawing on the evidence from the seminal Alameda County study in the USA, Berkman and Glass show that people who live in isolation from others, disconnected from people, are at increased risk of dying prematurely and 'this independently of health behaviours such as smoking, alcohol consumption, physical activity [and] preventive health care' (Berkman and Glass, 2000, p159). These authors also look at a wide variety of such studies and conclude that virtually all of them find that socially isolated people 'have between two to five times the risk of dying *from all causes* compared to those who maintain strong ties to friends, family and community' (p160).

So we are presented with a vivid image of people's health being supported (or not) by a tissue of interconnections with emotional, social contexts in a series of dynamic interactions. This helps us go way beyond the notion of health as simply the absence of disease.

Of course, few of the social determinants of health work in isolation: unemployment is often linked to low educational status, low status sometimes to low social cohesion, and so forth. 'Hierarchy' (already referred to) is a word that features largely in the studies of the social gradient's impact on health, and in the work of Sapolsky. Sapolsky and Spencer's (1997) work on primates is often quoted: this has demonstrated that 'animals with fewer social affiliations have the familiar pattern of reduced basal cortisol levels and attenuated stress responses associated with chronic anxiety' (Wilkinson, 1999, p262). In other words, we can demonstrate psychosocial pathways to do with hierarchies and social networks which mediate biological changes in animals; changes which impact negatively or positively on their health. Human beings, we may safely say, are no different. Social networks, the experience of feeling esteemed and valued, whether in the home or in interaction with one's social world, strengthen the body's immune system, as we have seen earlier, and so help the person resist disease. Potentially at least, this may add years to life.

Of course, the inverse is also true: *social exclusion* depletes the body's resistance to disease and undermines the health of those who experience it. As the WHO says of people experiencing different forms of social exclusion such as migrants and the mentally ill:

> *They are sometimes excluded from citizenship and often from opportunities for work and education. The racism, discrimination and hostility*

> *that they often face may harm their health ... Stigmatizing conditions*
> *such as mental illness, physical disability or diseases such as AIDS makes*
> *matters worse. People living on the streets, who may suffer a combina-*
> *tion of these problems, suffer the highest rates of premature death.*
>
> Wilkinson and Marmot (1998), pp11–12

In Australia the Aboriginal population has a much lower life expectancy than the rest of the nation (Australian Bureau of Statistics, 2003). This is a population which has been decimated by racism and social exclusion on a massive scale. It is difficult not to see the relevance of the general remarks of Berkman and Glass on social exclusion and premature ageing as applying clearly to this group of people: 'we speculate that social isolation, disintegration, and disconnectedness influence mortality and therefore longevity or life expectancy by influencing the rate of ageing of the organism' (Berkman and Glass, 2000, p151).

Work

The notion of stress, whether acute or chronic, underlies or is at least associated with many of the social determinants of health, including those factors clustering around the general notion of work. Employment and working conditions are important social determinants of health. Having no remunerative work when one wants it is bad for one's health. Enjoying the work we do, feeling that our contribution is adequately rewarded and appreciated, influences our health and well-being. It seems also that a sense of control over one's work helps a person stay healthy – this linking, of course, to what has been said about hierarchies. This link between perceived control over one's working conditions and one's health is supported by the famous Whitehall study of English bureaucrats after ten and twenty-five-year follow-ups of this population:

> *... smoking, cholesterol, blood pressure, sedentary lifestyle, and height*
> *explain no more than a third of the gradient in coronary heart disease*
> *mortality. Our evidence from the Whitehall II study is that the psychoso-*
> *cial work environment, in particular low control, may make an impor-*
> *tant contribution to accounting for the gradient in coronary heart disease.*
>
> Marmot (2000), p363

The understanding of the role of sense of control in supporting good health is quite developed and the words 'active' and 'passive' feature in the literature. Where there is a sense of some general control over one's work context, 'the worker has been given more resources to cope with high psychological demands because he/she can make relevant decisions, such as planning working hours according to his/her own biological rhythm … facilitating feeling of mastery and control in unforeseen situations', whereas the opposite, lack of control, the *passive* situation, 'may be associated with loss of skills and to some extent psychological atrophy' (Theorell, 2000, p98).

Culture

Another dimension of the context or environment of people that impacts, sometimes massively, on their health, is what we can call their 'culture': the value system shared and in a variety of ways imposed on people as the 'norm' in terms of relationships and interaction with society. Culture has to do with the way people see their world, the influence on their daily lives in the community in which they live. Culture, including religion, influences people's sense of self and worth, which we now know to be of considerable importance in maintaining people's health. We do not have to create rituals of conduct between members of families, 'elders' and so forth; we inherit and receive from our cultural context all kinds of modes of behaviour, mental maps which tell us how to act in many situations. The very stability this brings with it can often be good for one's health, and severe cultural disruption resulting in an individual not knowing how to act or how to interpret such taken-for-granted phenomena as body language can cause considerable stress and wear down the immune system.

A SNOWBALL OF FACTORS

Of course, as has been said, all of these factors interrelate in many ways. Both positively and negatively the social determinants of health interact on one another and on the health status of the people involved. Mention has been made already of biomedicine's

tendency to look for what is called 'specific aetiology', to seek to iso-
late as far as possible a single, generally biological, source of particular illnesses. Such a view, understandably, is resistant to the complexities provided by the work on the social determinants of health,
which helps us acknowledge that health – and illness – can be
'caused' by a multiplicity of factors, biological, social and emotional.

The research on social determinants of health does not completely invalidate exhortations in the direction of 'brown bread and
jogging' but it certainly helps relativize them while attesting to the
danger of reductionism inherent in simplistic versions of the
behavioural change approach to improving health status. The work
on the interaction between one's life context and capacity to engage
in lifestyle behavioural change is important here since yet again it
should breed caution in those who attempt to decontextualize
exhortations to people to 'improve their health'. The message of
this work on social determinants of health for all of us, lay people
and health professionals alike, is that biology and health services
and 'health promotion' strategies aimed at lifestyle are only part of
the improvement of the human health condition. The overwhelmingly important factors in maintaining health – and illness – lie in
the social fabric, the environment. The slogan must be, 'Think
health, think environment'. Environment of course must mean
more than the physical context and include the social, cultural,
emotional and economic context of people's lives, and also, as we
have said, appropriate and accessible health services.

We must see health as lying in the dynamic interaction between
the person and the environment in which they are situated. Other
cultures have had a keener understanding of health in this sense,
and it is to several of these that we shall turn in the next chapter.

4

LEARNING FROM OTHER CULTURES: HEALTH AS THE FIT BETWEEN THE PERSON AND THEIR ENVIRONMENT

The continued existence or otherwise of all creatures is dependent on the proper, inadequate, excessive or wrong interaction between them and their environmental factors.
Caraka Samhita, early Indian medical text (see below), commentary on Car. Sutra 11–44. Shree Gulabkunverba Ayurvedic Society (1949), p542

This chapter draws on the insights of non-western health cultures that reinforce the case for a model of health – and health care – which moves us beyond the limitations of the more static and segregated approach common in the west. There is a sense of health as interaction with the total environment in many non-western health cultures which can cast light on the model of health being developed.

HEALTH AS BALANCE IN NON-WESTERN HEALTH CARE SYSTEMS

It is one of the ironies of our times that many people in the western world, including many health professionals, are seeking to acquire a more dynamic and contextualized view of health by learning from eastern wisdom at the very time when many people in Asian cultures seem to be rushing to westernize their social systems, including their health care systems, as fast as possible. This cultural expansion of western systems, wrapped as they are in their own philosophical positions and therefore values, has been dubbed *cultural invasion*. It is most obvious in the proliferation throughout the world of fast-food outlets featuring items of dubious nutritional value such as hamburgers, disturbing, even if not replacing, long-held traditions of eating often solidly based in nutritional wisdom. The same phenomenon is manifest also in health systems – what has been called the 'McDonaldisation' of health care (Ritzer, 2000) – in the spread of western health culture. This takes the form of systems (rather like a global franchise) focused on curative care based in hospitals featuring expensively trained personnel using costly high-tech equipment. So, to repeat, we have largely decontextualized health care systems with very little emphasis on the maintenance of health and well-being and a high emphasis on delivery of treatment at tertiary level. With this phenomenon of globalization of systems and their underpinning values there is inevitably a weakening of other indigenous traditions which, though they might have considerable things to learn from the west, risk to lose that very thing which the west seems to lack: a health culture of wholeness in which human health is conceived as a dynamic balance with one's environment.

Health as environment, or rather, the dealing with the environment, is often a central notion in non-western societies. Many of the great eastern traditions of health care, including the Chinese and the Indian, in addition to dealing with illness as it presents itself, have the notion of the creative encounter with the environment – personal, social and physical – built into their systems of thought and practice. In our time western people are drawing from these traditions in piecemeal ways; for example, attempting to incorporate acupuncture or some techniques of yoga or Ayurvedic medicine into western ways of thinking and doing. A deeper understanding of these health care systems is now called for, a new synthesis. This will not be found in this book, but I will draw on what I understand of the eastern traditions' ideas of health as the dynamic interaction between individuals and communities and their total environment in order to argue the case for a broadening of our conceptual framework of health and therefore health systems. It is not insignificant that I am writing in Australia, a country sitting on the edge of Asia which, at the time of writing, is deeply involved in a sometimes ambivalent contact with the populations of this continent and their cultures. There is much to learn from these traditions, much that can free westerners from non-productive and reductionist mindsets concerning health and health care. The Australian Aboriginal culture itself, although this population has suffered the enormous trauma of colonization and displacement, both physical and cultural, has within it a dynamic understanding of health as wholeness which may yet in an ironic way benefit the descendants of the colonizers.

> *Western medicine is primarily interested in the recognition and treatment of disease. Traditional medicine seeks to provide meaningful explanation for illness and to respond to the personal, family and community issues surrounding illness. Traditional medicine explains not only the 'how' but also the 'why' of sickness.*
>
> *The Aboriginal approach to health care is a holistic one. It recognises the social, physical and spiritual dimensions of health and life. Their concept of health in many ways is closer than that of Western medicine to the WHO definition of health, 'a state of complete physical, mental and social well being and not merely the absence of disease or infirmity'.*
>
> Devanesen (2000), p1

THE CHINESE MEDICAL SYSTEM

It is impossible to do justice in such a short space to the wisdom of Chinese medicine or offer a comprehensive critical analysis of its impact on western ways of thinking and doing health care. Nor could the present writer attempt such a task. But there is plenty of evidence that in our time we are witnessing in the contact between 'western' and Asian health care systems a challenge to the limitations of western ways of conceptualizing and practising medicine (New Health Digest, 2004). The first step has often been the breaking down of some prejudices about these 'eastern' health systems. Contact with a variety of powerful and sometimes clearly effective, but different, ways of dealing with health has brought about a certain opening to learn on the part of some western people, both lay and professional, involving a way of revisiting what we think we know.

> *Treating headache by placing pins in the hands or treating asthma by placing needles in the feet challenges modern biomedical understanding.*

Thirty years ago, most physicians considered acupuncture a Chinese equivalent of voodoo. Despite the strangeness of its theory and method, in a very short period, acupuncture has changed from a cultural curiosity to an alternative therapy that, at a minimum, deserves a respectful hearing.

Kaptchuk (2002), p374

Ted Kaptchuk, a practitioner of Chinese medicine living in the US, says 'one of the important lessons I learned was that much of what we think is extraordinary in another place is just the ordinary not understood or experienced' (Kaptchuk, 2000, pxxi).

Historically, western medicine has been much influenced by its doctrine of 'specific aetiology' – the tracing of a clinical symptom back to a single major cause (Macdonald, 2000). This is part of the culture of dualism, the reductionist attempt to separate out the complex mind–body phenomena inherent in human life. 'The Chinese physician, in contrast, directs his or her attention to the complete physiological and psychological individual' (Kaptchuk, 2000, p4). In this way, simplistic single lines of causality are seen as inappropriate and Chinese practitioners are quite at ease with the notion of *co-morbidity*, which is increasingly recognized in western practice (McCabe and Holmwood, 2002). It is not only from the Chinese or Indian traditions that people in the west are seeking more satisfactory and less reductionist explanations of health and illness and therefore different therapies: for many people dissatisfied with 'allopathic' medicine one of the attractions of alternative therapies like homeopathy and naturopathy is that these practitioners and other alternative and traditional therapists tend also to see the patient in a more holistic context. There is, however, a kind of 'holism' growing in the west which would confine its vision of the 'whole' to the health of individuals seen in isolation, again making abstract from the socio-political dimensions of the context. Both the work on the social determinants of health dealt with in the last chapter and the broad view of the eastern tradition would go beyond this narrow view of what constitutes 'whole'.

At the basis of Chinese medicine are Taoist or Confucian philosophy and the concept of Yin-Yang, two polar complements of total reality. Yin and Yang 'represent a way of thinking. In this system of thought, all things are seen as part of a whole' (Kaptchuk, 2000, p8).

Comparing East and West, Kaptchuk sees the difference in this way: western thought is preoccupied with cause and effect and is based on the foundation of ideas of a *creator*. Chinese thought, in Taoism, on the other hand, is concerned with 'insight into the web of phenomena, not the weaver' (ibid., p15). Health, in Chinese thinking, is a state of *harmony* and disease a state of *disharmony*. In the lead-up to the declaration of Primary Health Care (PHC) at Alma Ata, the World Health Organization was struggling with the inadequacies of the western 'medical' model to meet the health needs of many countries and showed some interest in the experience of the 'barefoot doctor' – revolutionary China's (often successful) attempt to create a cadre of workers closer to the community and more affordable than a western-type doctor. The enthusiastic endorsement of the Chinese experience has been criticized as being somewhat simplistic and certainly it would be naïve to even suggest a simple transfer of the Chinese thinking and practice to other contexts. The point being made here, however, is that despite this, it is undeniable that in Chinese thinking there is an underlying vision of health as well-being, a balance, a notion which is not actively present in what we have called the western 'medical model'. PHC approaches have other things in common with Chinese health philosophy. 'Chinese medicine offers a different vision of health and disease, one that is implicitly critical of Western medicine because it refuses to see the individual as an entity separate from his or her environment' (Kaptchuk, 2000, p258). PHC approaches have held on to a similar philosophy without the back-up of a holistic health philosophy as in China and swimming against the mainstream of the western philosophy behind western medicine which separates the mind and the body in an artificial way.

We watch with interest as China comes into greater contact with western ideas and interests. Whatever synthesis between Chinese and western medicine is achieved will have important consequences for our emerging global health culture.

AYURVEDIC MEDICINE

It is a remarkable achievement that the Ayurvedic health system, 'traditional Indian medicine' with a long recorded experience, has survived at all in India. Given the impact of colonialism and its inevitable superiority complex towards all that is indigenous, one might have expected the ancient traditional health science to have survived only in folk form in rural areas. The reality is more complex. Folk versions do still persist, but Ayurvedic schools of medicine have also survived, albeit often seen, even by Indian people themselves, as poor cousins of the 'real thing', the system of health care practised by their western allopathic counterparts.

Ayurveda has survived, both formally as a science preserved and taught in Ayurvedic universities, as well as in the popular culture of India. It has important insights for us as we try to find ways of building health and not just disease systems and of conceptualizing health as a dynamic relationship between the person and their environment.

> *Ayurveda is primarily the science of positive health and it is only secondarily that it is the science for the cure of disease.*
> Shree Gulabkunverba Ayurvedic Society (1949), p247

The Ayurvedic medical philosophy is one of combining treatment with the promotion of health: in the words of the *Caraka Samhita*, a very ancient Indian medical text: 'Now, medicine is of two kinds: one kind is promotive of vigour in the healthy, the other destructive of disease in the ailing' (ibid., p624).

We have spoken of the usefulness and limitations of the analogy of the body as a machine, the mindset of western medicine. Ayurveda is quite clear of the danger of a too simplistic analogy:

> *The human body is no doubt a machine but the metaphor should be applied in a limited sense only. Even as a machine it is (a) self-stoking, self-adjusting, self-repairing, self-preserving, self-asserting and self-multiplying machine. It has intelligence and feeling. It has individuality and purposiveness. It is an organism much beyond the concept of mechanism ... Unlike western medicine, the focus on health rather than disease remains paramount, one of its basic tenets being the strengthening of 'the vital force of life to counteract the effect of wear and tear'.*
> (ibid.), pp247–249

Of course, we are talking philosophy here, not in any abstract sense, without reference to daily life, but rather acknowledging that it is impossible to talk health without situating that 'discourse' in the cultural context of a given population. An important part of any given cultural context is the conception that the people who live and breathe that culture have of their interaction with the world around them. This is a major difficulty in seeking to change popular and professional culture regarding health. The Anglo-Saxon culture which has come to dominate the forces of globalization is not a culture with an explicit philosophy of the self, certainly not of the self as a being essentially in interaction with itself and its environment. In the philosophical desert inhabited by most of us in the west, the pervasive though implicit philosophy of the self would have us see human society as an aggregate of consuming individuals and the human being perhaps, as *Homo economicus*. Western values, as Pickering (2001) tells us, '... create desires wherever they go and the fulfilment of those desires becomes central to wellbeing' (p2).

In contrast, speaking of the philosophy underpinning Ayurvedic medicine, our Indian commentator of the 1940s has this to say:

> *Man* [sic] *was studied in his whole personality which is the dynamic organisation within the individual of those psycho-physical systems that determine his unique adjustment to his environment, and the authors of Ayurveda, 'The Science of Life', intended by Ayurveda much more than mere skill of treatment or diagnosis of a diverse condition. It meant for them the total concept of life which includes man and his environment. The well-being of man, the aggregate of body, mind and soul, cannot be confined to mere physical health, but extends to that total sense of enjoyment of physical, mental and spiritual satisfaction and enrichment born as a result of wholesome and mutually beneficial interaction between the individual and his environment, social, physical and spiritual. Man as a biological entity needs to adjust to the physical environment and as a social and spiritual entity needs to adjust to the society in which he lives and to the spiritual ideal upheld by it. Such-well being alone is real and true of man in his entirety and such is the object of the 'Science of Life'.*
> Shree Gulabkunverba Ayurvedic Society (1949), pp525–526

It seems to me that the above text not only carries within it insights into Indian understanding of health but is resonant with many insights which we have discovered in western health science in recent years. It is a profoundly modern text. In the eastern context, then, health as interaction with one's total environment is a concept underpinning all medical culture. Slowly in the west we are coming to a similar understanding and we experience the difficulty of taking this on board in a holistic and 'natural' way. In much eastern philosophy of health it is obvious that health is about this positive engagement with the whole of one's environment:

> *For the medical sciences particularly, life goes always with its environment. Every organism and specially man must be understood always in relation to his environment, for all his life-functions are engrossed in a continual flux to meet the challenge or reap the benefit of the factors of the environment ... Caraka expresses this truth as a philosophical axiom that is the existence of all beings is derived from the nature of their reaction to environment.*
> Shree Gulabkunverba Ayurvedic Society (1949)

The unnamed commentator in the above text from the 1940s goes on to quote a phrase from the ancient Ayurvedic manuscript itself which explains the phenomenon of health in ways that we can see to be thoroughly modern and supported by much of the research of the social determinants of health: 'The continued existence or otherwise of all creatures is dependent on the proper, inadequate, excessive or wrong interaction between them and their environmental factors' (Commentary on Car. Sutra 11–44, ibid., p542).

The idea of all our 'life-functions' being engrossed in a continual flux to meet the challenge or reap the benefits of the factors of the environment is totally at one with our present day understanding of 'social biology' and health as the management of one's social determinants.

So, while the west was developing its own remarkable health and medical culture and yet, in certain areas at least, beginning to acknowledge the limitations of its reductionist approaches, other cultures, as in China or India (and not only there, of course), were in possession of broader visions and practices, waiting to be shared and to 'complement' the western view. Humility would, yet again, be of considerable use to us here.

5
RECONCEPTUALIZING HEALTH

Despite nearly two decades of repeated intellectual efforts to redirect health policy away from curative medicine to more fundamental interventions, the task remains largely undone. Why? ... Health policies at any time reflect the prevailing conceptions of what health is ... Ergo, any significant policy change requires the modification of a nations' underlying belief system — what intellectual historians would regard as the prevailing health paradigm.

Evans et al (1994), pp218–219

Health is the outcome of the quality of the person-environment fit.

Grzywacz and Fuqua (2000), p1

Throughout this work the suggestion has been that conventional western ways of thinking about health miss the complexities of the health phenomenon, both in its manifestations in individuals, and in our capacity as a society to foster health and manage illness. The need for more fruitful ways of understanding health and building health systems more responsive to human need has been becoming more evident by the year. The discussion in an earlier chapter of Primary Health Care highlighted the need for a new way of thinking about health and therefore health care since that story illustrates a significant frustration on the part of many people with the results of conventional thinking about health. Put crudely (but accurately), reductionist views of health have led to sometimes grotesque imbalances in health systems with institutions of care concerning themselves principally with disease and not with health. Attention has been drawn to the decontextualization of health in western practice and the alternative views inherent in non-western health systems, as well as to the growing evidence of the centrality of context to many conditions of health and illness. This chapter sets out to draw these ideas together and ask, in the light of the discussion of the preceding chapters: can we take a further step towards finding a way of conceptualizing health which leads us forward?

The obvious question: *what then, is health?* must be asked – the simple, straightforward question that never really gets addressed or risks dismissal as silly, theoretical or a waste of time. Yet it is arguably because we have not had the courage to ask this basic question and look for modern answers to it that we lack the capacity to create health systems that are truly responsive to populations and the individuals in them. We have allowed those with vested interests (often market-based) in promoting the glamour and promises of technical medical interventions, including the pharmaceutical companies, to shape our thinking and practice of health care.

The literature on social determinants, with its deepening understanding of the role of *context* in the health phenomenon, has been highlighted, although only touched on, as a pointer towards more fruitful ways of thinking and 'doing' health. Attention has been drawn to other pointers from non-western cultures.

The famous definition of health that the WHO espoused in the last century has been a constant reminder of the need to keep a broad view of health:

> *Health is the total physical, psychological and social well-being of individuals and communities and not merely the absence of disease.*

Despite this attempt by the WHO to remind us of the need for a holistic view of health, 'health systems' continue to be, as we have said, by and large, *medical* systems. Health, to a large extent, is encouraged or threatened by the environment in which we live. Or more accurately, it is a product of the person's interaction, for good or ill, with that environment. A new synthesis emerges from a consideration of health as this engagement or interaction and we are led to a new way of thinking and therefore of planning and implementing health systems.

THE CONTRIBUTION OF 'SALUTOGENESIS'

As has been said, western health systems are straining to be contained within a model in which the main focus is the health professional acting upon a decontextualized, needy or unwell, passive individual. Equally inadequate in terms of the role of context is the notion of health as being principally a matter of individual responsibility: the person 'taking charge' of the factors affecting their health. We need a way of thinking – and acting – about health that sees the well-being of a person as a process in which that person interacts dynamically with their total environment: their physical, emotional and social contexts. Some parts of this environment can be controlled or manipulated to an extent by the individual, and health-promotion messages often focus on these: smoking and safe sex are examples of this domain. Other dimensions of the environment, as in the case of living in a heavily polluted or illegally occupied country, lie outside the individual's immediate control but impact nevertheless, often very seriously, on health.

In the framework of health as interaction with the total environment, the professionals are often called upon to see themselves in a much more humble light than has been the case heretofore. The professional becomes facilitator of that process of positive interaction with or recovery from negative interaction with the environment. This is the case even in the most dramatic of interventionist surgery where the surgeon removes and even replaces a part of the body. The difference between operating on a cadaver and on a living person is surely that the living person's body reacts after the operation to rebuild tissue. Likewise, antibiotics work to remove certain bacteria to give space for healing to take place; the body has to revitalize itself. In both cases it is the life force of the human body which is being encouraged to come into play and engage in the process of healing, even if this essential dynamic dimension is not sufficiently recognized in westernized medical cultures. The same must be said of interventions in mental health: their purpose is surely to allow the human spirit to manage its environment more successfully.

And here we run into the problem of language. Language shapes our way of seeing the world and is, in turn, shaped by it. In the case of health and health services, language can shape policies and practice. The words 'life force engaging with its environment' do not trip off the tongue easily, at least in English. Health as the dynamic between the energy of an individual and his or her context in the way we have described is not a difficult concept to grasp, but the words to describe it convincingly can fail us or sound strange. To indicate that sense of the agency of the person dealing with their context, I will use the words 'life force' until someone finds a more acceptable term. I see the words 'life force' and 'health' as inter-changeable, although some might be happier with the more passive notion of health and see it as the result of the interaction between the life force and the environment.

Health, then, should be seen as the dynamic interaction between this life force of human beings and their environment. A simple vocabulary check can be useful here: if we want to complement the clinical preoccupation with disease and pathologies, we need a vocabulary that will convey this more comprehensive and dynamic dimension, we need words as a vehicle for the enormous cultural shift involved to get the public and professionals thinking *health*. Ideally, this would encourage a preoccupation with the creation of environments that foster health being built into planning and resource allocation in health systems. However, the fact is – for reasons we have elaborated – that the vocabulary in health care circles in general has largely to do with disease and other pathogenic concerns: 'at-risk conditions' and the 'fixing up' of these problems. If we wish to think and talk and plan *health* and not just the management of *disease*, we need a vocabulary, a way of conceptualizing this emphasis. We can ask ourselves: what is the opposite of *pathologies* and *pathogenic*? The words do not spring too easily to our lips. We see what we are trained to look for, what our globalized so-called 'health' culture disposes us to look for, and as it stands it is: illness, disease, the pathological and how to prevent or avoid it.

The idea of salutogenesis can help here. The word is borrowed from Antonovsky (1987, 1988, 1996) and its meaning expanded. *Salutogenesis* means simply the creation or formation or origins of *health*, in contradistinction to *pathogenesis*, the creation or origins of *disease*. If salutogenesis seems a strange word to some, this is at least in part a reflection of our western 'health' system's preoccupation with illness and what is broken. This pathological orientation is part of the more general culture and is reflected in language; we have words for disease processes and not for health generation. Even the non-specialist is used to the negative dimension of the health vocabulary: 'pathological' is a common enough term. It is surely significant that words do not come easily, either to health professionals or the general public, when they are asked to describe what is happening in the process of healing or to name the oppo-site of 'pathological' or 'pathogenic'. This is why the translations from the eastern medical cultures which do reflect this more dynamic understanding seem strange to the western mind. 'Vital force' seems alien. Suggestions such as 'health-promoting' or 'health-enhancing' are sometimes offered, but somehow they seem less than convincing, failing to match or counteract the vigour of the vocabulary for the negative. This is especially true of the medical profession, which is trained to think in terms of the treatment of illness. This is an important but partial dimension of planning any health system, whether a family's, a community's or a country's. We need words to reflect our understanding of the strength of the dynamic life force which is the health of the person.

Antonovsky was preoccupied by the capacity of some human beings to deal with even the most negative and hostile forces in their environment in a vigorous manner which resulted in the enrichment of the person rather than their diminishment. He had a major interest in those people who had survived the experience of internment at the time of the Holocaust. He marvelled that some people, far from being crushed by the horrors of the environment thrust upon them and the consequent humiliations they had to endure, had actually been enriched as human beings; they had interacted with their apparently totally destructive environment in a way which, astonishingly, nourished their inner selves. Their spirits had not only triumphed over adversity, but flourished. This led him to coin the term 'salutogenesis':

> *A pathological orientation seeks to explain why people get sick, why they enter a given disease category. A salutogenic orientation (which focuses on the origins of health) poses a radically different question: why are people located towards the positive end of the health ease/disease continuum, or why do they move towards this end, whatever their location at any given time.*
>
> Antonovsky (1987), ppxii–xiii

For Antonovsky, the interest is in the psychological orientation of the individual which leads them to believe that they can make the most of the situation:

> *The answer to the salutogenic question that I developed was the sense of coherence concept (SOC) … a global orientation that expresses the*

extent to which one has a pervasive, enduring though dynamic, feel-
ing of confidence that one's internal and external environments are
predictable and that there is a high probability that things will work
out as well as can reasonably be expected.

(ibid.), ppxii–xiii

Antonovsky's orientation is similar to that of a psychologist: he looks to the individual's response to situations to better understand their feelings and their reactions. Specifically, he is interested in the characteristics of the individual psyche, the 'sense of coher-ence', which enable *this* individual to cope in circumstance where others would not. I feel that his insights are extremely enlighten-ing and useful in helping us understand what some call *resilience* and how different people react differently under stress. The con-tribution of Antonovsky and, explicitly, of his thinking on saluto-genesis, has been acknowledged in Germany more than in other countries, taking up his ideas on *sense of coherence* as part of the explanation of how some people's coping with potential disease stressors differs from other people's (Bengel et al, 1999).

Implicit to this notion of salutogenesis is the idea of a positive activity on the part of the individual as he/she engages with their environment: though Antonovsky wouldn't use these words, it is entirely consistent with his insights to suggest that his notion of health is the positive interaction of the human life force with its environment.

A pathological or, strictly speaking, a pathogenic orientation seeks to see what the factors are in the person's social, economic and emo-tional environment which generate or foster the growth of illness and malfunction. As we have said, this preoccupation with the nega-tive has dominated western medicine, including the discipline of psy-chology. There are, however, signs of change in that culture:

For years, nested within an 'illness model' of psychology, researchers
have searched for the sources or antecedents of negative outcomes.
There has been a neglect of the roots of the field of psychology –
normative behavioural processes. Only recently have we turned
toward a model based more on health than on illness, and only recent-
ly have we recognized that in order to effectively study deviations in
behaviour, or abnormality, we must also have a more clearly defined

concept of what normal or healthy means and understand the origins of health – 'salutogenesis'. Accompanying this focus upon health-related processes has been the conceptualization of 'resilience' or 'invulnerability', together with the new investigations of antecedents and correlates of resilient development.

Hauser et al (1989), p111

The notion of resilience takes us some of the way towards a more dynamic understanding of health, but for people examining the phenomenon of resilience, the focus is still on dealing with the hard blows, the management of the difficult in the environment. 'Salutogenesis' potentially encompasses this but would include also being nourished by the positive in the environment. The word allows for the process of engagement with those things in the environment that foster health, that nourish wellness. This is in line with the Indian Ayurvedic text we have seen in which health is understood as the ability to interact positively with one's milieu or context: *We are in a continual flux to meet the challenge or reap the benefit of the factors of the environment.*

A concern with salutogenesis, a salutogenic preoccupation, can go beyond an understanding of individual psychology, in this case the capacity of individuals to make good out of bad. It can help us imagine health as being a process, a dynamic, an engagement by which we 'reap the benefits' of the environment. Just as a pathogenic orientation indicates a concern with the origins of disease, the making of disease, so a salutogenic preoccupation can convey a concern with the origins of wellness or health: health as the creation of well-being, through engagement with the environment. And these environments, when they foster this well-being can be seen as 'salutogenic'.

I suggest that both senses of 'salutogenic' are very helpful to us as we look for a more useful model of health: the salutogenic perspective on the individual person as he/she interacts with their environment (both to deal with phenomena which threaten balance and to absorb support from phenomena which nourish the 'life force') and the concern to foster salutogenic environments, environments that facilitate the growth and maintenance of health in individuals and communities.

Although the terminology may be unfamiliar, this broadening of the individual biological and psychological focus to include wider social perspectives and contexts known to be crucial to the creation and maintenance of health in individuals and communities has, of course, characterized other health work in the community; saluto-genesis simply seeks to name this phenomenon.

We are moving away from the model of a health system that would see the passive individual or community being acted on by the health professional when individuals have failed to take proper care of their health, or 'fallen ill', towards a model in which the health professional witnesses and where possible facilitates the capacity of the individual or community to interact positively with the environment and the building up of the environment that fosters such growth. Of course, this is altogether a more humble approach to the process of healing and maintenance of health than we have seen heretofore in western medicine.

Often in common speech we do not distinguish enough between health and health care, as in 'Departments of Health' or 'I work in health'. Thinking of salutogenesis and salutogenic environments allows us to better distinguish them: *health*, the dynamic interaction of the individual with the environment, and *health care*, the actions undertaken (by whoever) to facilitate that process of inter-action with the biological and social environment.

HEALTH AS POSITIVE INTERACTION WITH THE ENVIRONMENT

Common sense and a reflection on the practice of daily living and a humble openness to the health-related wisdom of non-western cultures support the idea that health is about the interaction between a person or a group and their context, their environment. In family groupings that are more or less functional, health is understood, at least implicitly, as interacting with the environment, as managing the context. It is a matter of concern that western culture is now much more preoccupied with family breakdown, with the pathologies of families, with the *pathogenic*, than with all those processes that occur in most families which are health enhancing, *salutogenic.* Our culture seems obsessed with its failures, encouraging parents to focus, for example, on their bad parenting and its origins – perhaps their own experience of bad parenting – rather than being concerned with the acknowledgement of and the supporting and building on the myriad positive, health-enhancing, salutogenic phenomena that are present in the daily life of most families. In families in general there is a concern to enable family members, especially the children, to deal with what is bad or threatening in the social-economic, cultural context in which they find themselves as well as to be enriched and strengthened by what is positive – or salutogenic – in the environment. Often the focus is on dealing with and even being nourished by these environments. The 'health' dynamic is in both aspects, and has negative and positive dimensions: dealing with the hostile without being too 'unbalanced' by it and being nourished by the positive, whether physical or spiritual. The family context itself is, of course, part of this environment and contains both negative 'stressors' to be dealt with as well as positive, health-enhancing factors. In usual situations, the latter outweigh the former. The process of dealing well with both negative and positive can be seen as a salutogenic engagement with the environment. And that is what health is, this management of the environment. The efforts of the family members to create a supportive context for the physical, psychological and spiritual well-being of that family can be seen to be the creation of a salutogenic environment or milieu, facilitating the positive interaction.

Having said that, I invoke here the reader's recollections of a relatively functional family containing two, three or more members. I suggest that a look at this group of people, bound by blood or other personal ties, can help us understand what health is and what a health system should be, in terms of its essential components, but also suggest what is distorted about and missing from conventional western ways of thinking about health and building institutionalized health systems.

To begin with, a family functioning moderately well integrates treatment and prevention, mental and physical health. For example, a child returns home with a cut leg. Another family member, often a parent, cares for the cut. The wound is treated and the child is consoled. The child is seen as a whole human being, hurting on the 'outside and inside'. Often in such a domestic scenario as the one we describe, prevention is combined with the tending of the wound, with some communication about the need to avoid dangerous situations in the future. If the child is lucky, this part of the process is not just a telling off, but an assurance that she or he will be all right and still be cared for if another mishap does occur.

The potential outside negative impact is not, of course, only physical: the bullying that children experience is often psychological, affecting their spiritual self. Again, hopefully, the home offers a place where self-esteem can be reaffirmed and self-worth and confidence restored. Every parent knows that the health of their child is not only a matter of helping the child deal with disease or adversity but also involves the child being nourished physically and emotionally. To a large extent, the role of parents and others involved in children's development, like teachers, involves the dual role of encouraging the salutogenesis of the child, its ability to deal with the environment and the fostering of a salutogenic environment which can nourish his or her physical, emotional and spiritual dimensions. Sometimes this is an explicitly conscious salutogenic approach on the part of the parent or other adult, as in reassuring the child of their worth after occasions that challenge this. But there is a myriad of salutogenic activities going on which are often largely ignored, not least because of the focus on the pathological which I have already referred to as part of the general health/medical and child development culture of the end of the 20th century. On a daily basis children encounter acts of support and love from their parents as these busy themselves with what we could call the ecology of the healthy home: acts of protection, of physical and emotional nourishment, acts of love. The lucky ones experience different but also important respectful interactions from their teachers at school. It is well known that children, even if materially well cared for, who lack the salutogenic environment of love will fail to thrive and risk growing with damage to their emotional and spiritual selves, like abandoned children, or those who have been tragically separated from their parents, such as the Stolen Generation of Australian Aboriginal children (Aboriginal children forcefully removed from their families of birth and 'adopted' by white families with a view to incorporating them into the white society) (Human Rights and Equal Opportunity Commission, 1997). The tragedy in such cases is not only explicitly pathogenic influences – physical, sexual abuse – but the loss of the 'normal' salutogenic environment of the family as I have described it.

This 'family health system' offers its members, especially the younger members, an environment protected from disease, where possible, and a place where recovery is fostered when necessary. Such a system has, in addition to its pathological and pathogenic concerns, an equal concern with the conditions that foster and maintain well-being, what we can call a salutogenic preoccupation. In this way this 'non-professional' health system like the family is actually more balanced in its approach to health and illness: unlike the professional one, its *raison d'être* is not only to react to what is going wrong, to illness, but to foster health.

BIOLOGY PLUS

The notion of health as the *fit* between the person and his/her environment is, of course, not new, even in western thought; in the science of biology we have already a powerful model of health as the constant adaptation of the organism to the environment. Dubos reminded us as long ago as 1959 that, biologically speaking, health was the maintenance of *homeostasis*: the balance that organisms and organic systems manage to maintain between competing influences, both those which sustain and those which threaten in its environment (Dubos, 1970).

> *Homeostasis implies two separate, but interdependent, concepts. One recognises that the body can function well only if its milieu interieur remains within limits characteristic for each organism. The other acknowledges that the body must make rapid adjustments to correct for the disturbing effects of constantly changing external conditions. In principle, health can be maintained only if these two conditions are simultaneously satisfied through complex hormonal and biochemical processes governed by what Cannon picturesquely called the 'wisdom of the body'.*
>
> Dubos (1970), p93

Dubos was drawing on the work of authors such as Cannon, who seems to be the first to use the expression 'homeostasis'. He saw it as 'a condition – a condition which may vary, but which is relatively constant' (Cannon, 1932, p24). In his turn, Cannon was drawing on the work of earlier physiologists such as Charles Richet, who was intrigued by the stability/instability of the living being:

> *The living being is stable. It must be so in order not to be destroyed, dissolved or disintegrated by the colossal forces, often adverse, which surround it. It maintains its stability only if it is excitable and capable of modifying itself according to external stimuli and adjusting its response to the stimulation.*
>
> (quoted in Cannon, 1932, p21)

Adjustment is of the essence of this dynamic process of life itself.

I find it of note that the emphasis in both Cannon and Richet is on the forces which threaten life, which threaten to disintegrate it, rather than on the capacity to manage such adversity and an emphasis on whatever it is that promotes life and this ability to deal with adversity.

AN EXPANDED NOTION OF ENVIRONMENT

If we extend the notion of environment to include not just the physical environment but the social, cultural, economic and psychological and spiritual worlds of people, then the same axiom can apply: health is situated in the homeostasis to be maintained in all of these interacting worlds. The idea of health as homeostasis suggests a dynamic balance, not something static, at rest. This conveys the sense of health as a living process, a dealing with forces which either nourish life, are salutogenic (not a word used by Dubos) or threaten it (pathogenic, the entropy which Dubos speaks of). This simple idea of health as a dynamic balance seems to me to be the most useful way of thinking of health in keeping with our growing understanding not only of the complexities of the life of human beings but with our understanding of the need for an ecologically sound approach to our individual and collective lives. Andrew

Weil, in his book *Health and Healing*, gives us some insights into health conceived of in this way:

> *The balance of health is dynamic ... We are islands of change in a sea of change, subject to cycles of rest and activity, of secretion of hormones, and of the rise and fall of powerful drives, subjected to noise, irritants, agents of disease, electrical and magnetic fields, the deterioration of age, emotional tides. The variables are infinite and all is flux and motion. That equilibrium occurs even for an instant in such a system is miraculous, yet most of us are mostly healthy most of the time, our mind-bodies always trying to keep up the incredible balancing act demanded by all the stresses from inside and out.*
>
> Weil (1996), p51

ENGAGING WITH THE POSITIVE IN THE ENVIRONMENT

We could add that it would be useful to make explicit the positive in the environment that the living being encounters. As we have seen, we do not only encounter forces which threaten; we are healthy because we also encounter forces which nourish, which build, both physically and mentally and spiritually. Moreover, we need to see health not just as an individual's engagement with the world, but the interaction of communities and society with their environment. People find their balance as individuals but also as part of communities and society which both contribute to and are influenced by the larger world.

For many people an *ecological* perspective suggests concern for the natural and physical environment, an awareness of the need for the human species to respect and keep some balance with other life on this planet and preserve the human habitat as a fit place to live. But, given all we have said of the importance of all the contexts of human life and the inevitable interaction between these contexts (the personal with the social, with the political, etc.), it makes sense to widen the idea of *ecology*.

People with an ecological perspective on health are broadening our vision. As Daniel Stokols (2000) says

> *Many of the most vexing and enduring health problems ... are etiologically tied to a complex web of political, cultural, and economic conditions (p5).*

Social ecological analyses of health and illness are characterized by their broad contextual scope. That is, they examine health problems encountered by individuals and groups in relation to the etiologic circumstances present in their day-to-day physical and social environments (p1).

As we have said, the focus on most health care systems, certainly the western system, has been squarely on the pathogenic, that which is the bearer of illness. The attention, understandably no doubt, is riveted on what can go wrong; the preoccupation is with trying to 'fix' this and put it right. This has to be complemented by the salutogenic view, a focus on what bears health and wholeness, what builds. Just as biological science, as in Dubos' work, acknowledges the sustaining of life in the physical environment, so we should envisage health as the self dealing with the total environment, both physical and social, both that which is threatening in that environment and that which is sustaining. Homeostasis is achieved not only by engaging with the pathogenic, but equally as importantly, with that which is salutogenic, that which nourishes. It is the management of both which constitutes health.

Children cherished emotionally and well cared for materially in the early years of life are likely to have the resilience necessary to deal with negativity later on. It is obvious, surely, that the encounter with positive, constructive experiences is necessary to nourish what might be called *social homeostasis*.

Mental health is a good area to consider in terms of health a balance between destructive and enriching forces. Psychologists (professional and lay) know well that mental health is a balancing act. The mentally healthy person is one who deals with 'triumph and disaster'

If we extend the notion of environment to include not just the physical environment, embracing an expanded notion of ecology, to include the social, cultural, economic and psychological and spiritual worlds of people, then it is clear that health is the homeostasis to be maintained in all of these.

So, there is an environmental/ecological perspective to health at the level of biology: it can be seen as the dynamic equilibrium or homeostasis maintained by the body at an organic level. There is also an environmental/ecological dimension to health at the level of the person's conscious interaction with the widening circles of his/her encounters: the people, both family and friends, school, work, all of these are genuinely part of the 'environment' and the interaction with them either nourishes or threatens health. Health can be seen as the 'successful' interaction with all of these dimensions of the environment. There is also an environmental or ecological perspective to health at the community level: a healthy community would be one in which that community managed the circumstances of its environment in a similar way to the healthy organism, not being overcome by the pathogenic and taking nourishment and strength from the salutogenic.

Our growing understanding of the human immune system already referred to fits well within a framework of health as management of the environment, an ecology of health perspective. The immune system is precisely the mechanism in the individual human being which integrates the negative and the positive that the individual encounters.

Important in this regard is our growing knowledge of the mind-body unity already referred to: factors detrimental to our physical well-being impact also on our psychological well-being. But just as significantly, factors that impact positively on our mental well-being can impact positively on our immune system. The salutogenic influence of social support on the T-cells of the human immune system is an identifiable phenomenon (Williams, 2003).

In the whole area of mental health it is obvious, surely, that encounters with positive, constructive experiences, often play a crucial role in sustaining what might be called the process of *psychological homeostasis*.

Health, of course, is not 'environment' or ecological in any static sense: the mere juxtaposition of the physical, emotional and economic contexts or dimensions of individuals' lives. Rather, health can usefully be seen as the successful relationship that the individual or community has with this total environment, the dynamic balance or homeostasis in these environments, the ecological undertaking of the individual and the community and society. Individuals can often achieve a measure of balance with many dimensions of their contexts, personal, social, etc., and often 'health' messages are aimed at this dimension of the person–world interaction: look after your health. But a true ecological/environmental perspective recognizes that this is often the 'easy' part of the environment to exhort people about. Equally important, in various degrees, are the environments of job opportunities, discrimination, income distribution policies and a host of other factors which society is less keen to look at and over which the individual and even sometimes the community itself can do little about.

In other words, it is important to acknowledge, as both Weil and Antonovsky do, the positive force in the human being as he or she interacts with the environment, but it is also important to acknowledge and pursue and promote the salutogenic in the environment and, by implication, to denounce and eliminate the non-salutogenic in people's environments. I would argue that much of public and community health should be seen as the pursuit and creation of salutogenic environments for given populations.

I have argued elsewhere (Macdonald, 2000) that people's life context should be the focus of education about health rather than the present emphasis on lifestyle and personal behaviour. In a salutogenic perspective, health education is concerned with the strengthening of the person's (or community's) capacity to negotiate aspects of this environment, to forge a healthy ecology, personal and societal. What I am arguing for here is the extension of that simple idea. When environment and health are linked, the word 'environment' is generally reserved for the physical context, either 'natural' (for example, the weather and its impact on people's health) or artificial: the built environment, housing, etc. We must take a leap here and go beyond this notion of environment to include in it the social, cultural, economic and political environment. The challenging consequence of taking a truly 'holistic' approach to health is that there must be, at least potentially, room in our thinking for the 'whole'. In this way, we cannot understand the health of an individual or a community unless we think environment.

As we have seen, there has been a growing acknowledgment of the contribution of sectors other than the formal health sector to the maintenance of individual and community health. Unfortunately, the intersectoral collaboration for health called for since Alma Ata rarely occurs. However, if we conceptualize health and environment as being more closely linked than has generally been the case in western health systems, then I contend that there is much to be gained for the management of health in the lives of both individuals and communities.

It is not just that health workers should think environment. Environmentalists should think health: the notions of equity and participation, embedded in the policy documents promoting Primary Health Care, can challenge environmentalists by reminding them that, despite the horrors inflicted on our environment by human beings and a dominant anthropocentric ethos in development which has often been destructive and disrespectful of the physical environment, *people* are still an essential part of the environment. They, and particularly the disadvantaged and marginalized, must be a part of whatever equation is found to help us forward in the great ecological drama that is being played out in our time.

This expanded notion of environment has the potential to help health workers to break away from the limitations imposed by a narrow focus on the biophysical with patients as passive beneficiaries and to think and plan for health always in function of people's engagement with their total life context: their environment. What people work at, the very air they breathe, how they feel about themselves, what they eat, and a host of other contextual, *environmental*, dimensions of their lives are the very fabric of their health.

Lip service is often given to the need to draw together the two 'wings' of health care: the curative and the preventive. Dubos says this tension has profound historical roots, symbolized by the goddess Hygeia, who can be seen as representing the promotion of health and well-being, and her sister, Panacea, the treatment dimension (Dubos, 1970). The non-integration of these two dimensions of health systems is greater today than ever it was. We need an understanding of health care as a system, a whole, with less of a dualistic division between these two dimensions. A way out of this dualism is needed and can be found in this notion of engagement with the total environment. I would argue that a renewed notion of health, another way of thinking health, is called for, a view that sees health as being inextricably linked to environment (economic, cultural, social and personal as well as collective). This would need, in the first place, the re-orientation of health workers already referred to. So, I am not arguing for health workers, let us say for the moment, doctors and nurses, to simply acknowledge the importance of the physical environment for health and to endorse the work of those who work in this field. This could mean yet again an unnecessary Cartesian split as in 'we will do the health and you the environment'. Rather, I would argue that those health workers who could usually be categorized as health *care* workers should learn to *think* environment, to think of health *as* environment.

HEALTH IS ENVIRONMENT

The argument has been that health workers need to be helped to think of health in a new way and part of that thinking would involve an expanded notion of environment. Likewise, in the world of environmental management and environmental health there is a need for a concept of health that extends the notion of environment to include in it the people's access to basic health services. We need to include the notion of health care in our thinking about the environment. Often the separating out of environment and health care comes from a bureaucratic division of labour of professionals rather than from communities' perceptions. When communities are asked for their comments on improvement to their environment, these often would include some aspect of health service provision.

This is not to suggest that the only impediment to the reconceptualizing of health care and its consequent re-orientation lies in the attitudes and practices of the health profession. Fundamental orientations and the attitudes they engender are, however, a real part of what needs to be changed and hopefully health professional training is already moving towards an understanding of 'health is environment', even if only slowly. The interest in our time in 'social epidemiology' (Berkman and Kawachi, 2000) holds out hope in this regard. The discussion about the education of health professionals must surely include the debate as to whether this orientation towards an understanding of the social as well as the biological roots of health and illness should be left to postgraduate studies, as in Masters of Public Health courses. Surely the orientation towards health rather than illness, towards an understanding of the social determinants of health, must begin as early as possible in the training of all health professionals. As Lomas and Contandriopoulos (1994) say in the context of broadening the perceptions of the medical profession during their medical school training to incorporate ideas coming from research on the social determinants of health:

> Over the longer term, the key to changing the dominant belief systems in medicine lies in the medical school. Indeed, the present trend in medical education is to do just that by giving greater emphasis to, public and community health and other population-based views in the medical curriculum (p281).

Stressing the importance of education and training is not to deny that to change current thinking and practice around health and its maintenance requires more than a reworked medical curriculum. It is clear that the current emphasis on high-tech medicine, inevitably costly equipment and medication serves economic interests other than those of health professionals. The world of ideas, such as those in this book, can have little impact in changing vested economic interests in existing 'health' culture such as those of pharmaceutical corporations and those companies which manufacture the 'hardware' of the disease industry. A popular understanding of health and environment is required, community education on the grand scale. Inspired and informed political leadership would be called for.

Behind this criticism of the dominant culture of biomedicine and its influence on health policy is the hope that we can move towards a notion of environment that includes the social as well as the physical. The need for a new vision of health as environment is universal.

Health, then, is the successful relationship individuals and communities have with their environment.

On one level, such a remark is merely common sense and informs the work of many health care practitioners. It is clear, for example, that although an individual normally presents themselves for 'care' when experiencing some symptom of distress of dis-ease or illness, that condition has arisen out of a context, an environment, and the person with the condition, even though 'cured', will return to that environment and often to the risk of the same or similar illness. This is as true of 'diseases of poverty' as it is of 'diseases of affluence'. In the case of communicable diseases the logic is blindingly obvious. If workers in the health services, faced with such conditions as measles, scabies, lice or diarrhoea, focus only on the individual and his or her symptoms without acknowledging the need for change in their context, their environment, the condition will recur. Hence, of course, the need for a list of notifiable disease because of the threat to others. Such awareness is fundamental to health-system thinking and the growth of public health. But in western societies, too, there is need for a public health perspective in the work of all health workers and to extend the notion of 'environment' beyond the idea of disease vectors. The isolated pensioner with anxiety attacks or the isolated young mother of three with depression are being treated in a system which is geared to see and treat them in isolation from their context, yet their environment is just as interconnected with their 'health' as is that of the poor person in a context of communicable diseases.

Unfortunately, this notion of health as positive interaction with one's environment has rarely extended beyond the notion of 'controlling' biological contamination. We now know much more about the impact on health of other environments, less obvious (and often, of course, less easily controlled), but no less significant: people's social, cultural, economic, psychological and spiritual environment. Just as it is woefully inadequate to return a child rehabilitated from diarrhoea into the context or environment that gave rise to the problem in the first place, it is equally inappropriate to return someone with chronic depression, after medication, to the environment – social, familial, economic or whatever – that contributed to the condition in the first place.

More positively put, health is so embedded in the psychological, physical, social, cultural and spiritual environment that one can say: *health is environment*. Or, better: it is the successful interaction/relationship which individuals and communities have with their environment.

6

AN EXAMPLE – THE HEALTH OF MEN: A SALUTOGENIC APPROACH

The Doctors' Reform Society recognizes that there are particular issues for men which affect their health. These issues can arise from the process of socialization to compete and dominate in social and political spheres which can foster violence. As a result of this, many men experience a number of psychological difficulties, a reluctance to acknowledge and address their own health issues and diffidence in approaching health services.

Doctors' Reform Society Policy Statements (undated), Australia

(An example of a non-salutogenic approach to men's health.)

SUMMARY OF MODEL

It is not difficult to argue that men's health is a seriously neglected area of organized health care systems. The framework we have described allows us to rethink and plan for men's health; a salutogenic perspective can carry us forward here.

A salutogenic approach to the health of any population would involve both dimensions of the model we have outlined. First of all, it would acknowledge that health is the positive interaction with the total environment and that the capacity to do this must be encouraged. Then, in terms of populations, society must seek to provide a salutogenic environment to foster this interaction, the health of this population. As regards boys and men this perspective could be most useful. The argument for a fresh look at men's health is not a compensatory one, as in 'women's health has received some attention, so men's health should as well'. It is rather that in any population health approach one should adopt an overall systems look at the needs for prevention and access to care of different groups in their own right, whether children, women, older people or men. An objective view of the health needs and status of any population will lead to the inclusion of men's health issues as a matter of course. This has not always happened and even when it has, our view of men's health is to a large extent predetermined by the cultural perspectives we have on men. Some of these, it will be argued, have degenerated into the category of stereotypes and need to be challenged.

We have said in the previous chapter that a major characteristic of a salutogenic health approach would be the conceptualization of health that leads to a working model of health and health services which combines a balance between prevention and treatment, with an emphasis on *health* and its maintenance and not just on *disease* and its treatment. This can be seen as an encouragement of the process of salutogenesis in individuals and communities and the fostering of salutogenic environments.

The benefits of a salutogenic approach to men's health are considerable. One has only to look at the bulk of articles on 'men's health' to see the need for an approach that breaks new ground. The articles in academic journals dealing with men's health reflect an overwhelming concern with physical, psychological and social pathologies. Firstly, there are the articles dealing with tissues such as prostate and testicular cancer and such clearly male pathologies. Then there are the social pathologies, which we could describe as falling under the banner of 'men behaving badly'.

Many non-evidence-based assumptions continue to prevail in men's health. The discourse that has so far influenced policy development has tended to be in the mode of male deficiency: 'men don't take care of themselves', 'men don't go to the doctor', 'men are not in touch with their feelings', 'men don't communicate about their health'. To this already gloomy picture are added further stories about male deficiency: men and violence, and men as perpetrators.

A SALUTOGENIC APPROACH TO MEN'S HEALTH

The concern with testicular and prostate cancer and with coronary heart disease is, of course, laudable. But, interestingly, the literature on initiatives on men's health, even so-called 'health promotion' for men, has another major strand of concern: the social pathologies of men – men's violence, the prevention of abuse, the need to address men's inadequacies in 'talking about their emotions', men's failure to use health services, and so forth. It would seem to be accurate to talk of a 'deficit model' of men as underpinning this dimension of men's 'health'. Sometimes the physical pathologies – stroke, heart conditions and the like – are seen as flowing from the social pathologies, attributable to the phenomenon of 'men behaving badly'.

As an illustration of this, in one industrialized country, Australia, doctors who see themselves as progressive have formed the Doctors' Reform Society. Here is its Men's Health Policy:

8.3 Men's Health

8.3.1 *The DRS recognises that there are particular issues for men which affect their health. These issues can arise from the process of socialisation to compete and dominate in social and political spheres which can foster violence. As a result of this, many men experience a number of psychological difficulties, a reluctance to acknowledge and address their own health issues and diffidence in approaching health services. (see also 15. Violence and Aggression)*

8.3.2 *The DRS recognises that despite the fact that the majority of health research has been conducted on men and that there are biases towards men in health care teaching (due to the dominance of men in teaching and research positions), men still have poorer health in a number of areas and a lower life expectancy than women.*

8.3.3 *The DRS believes that increased attention to lifestyle changes (such as exercise, reduction of alcohol consumption, and strategies to reduce violence) are more important in improving the health of men than technological improvements in health care.*

8.3.4 *The DRS believes all men in Australia must have access to appropriate information and education about health. In particular, men need to be encouraged to make earlier, more appropriate use of primary health services.*

8.3.5 *The DRS encourages the development of accessible, appropriate services for those who are victims of violence. It is also important to develop preventive and treatment services for those who are at risk of, or have, perpetrated violence. (see also Violence and Aggression 15.1.3 General, 15.3 Domestic Violence and 15.4 Sexual Assault)*

8.3.6 *The DRS believes in order to improve men's health, the men's health movement needs to focus on the above issues, rather than competing with the women's health movement.*
  Doctors' Reform Society Policy Statements (undated), Australia

It is of note that in a policy of just over 250 words, *violence* is the most repeated word, mentioned seven times. This is a reflection of a culture stereotype: *men as violent, men as irresponsible* seems to be a preoccupation of some western health systems in their thinking and planning for men's health. Part of this 'deficit model' involves the notion that 'men don't go to the doctor enough or in time'. Of course, victims of male abuse and those who support them must inevitably be preoccupied with male violence. But what if I were a mother or father of boys and visited this website for insights into what was good for the health of my sons? Or a family interested in the well-being of a father after prostate surgery (a common concern)? Or a young doctor or psychologist looking to help my practice adopt a population health approach to all my clients, including men? To make a health service male-friendly? I would hardly find much help in such an approach.

The above is an excellent example of a non-salutogenic approach to men's health. A salutogenic approach would involve a radical change of perspective, not to say a sea change. In the first place, the concern would be to encourage the salutogenic *in* men: their ability to deal with the hostile and absorb the good in their environment. In a world where young men kill themselves with alarming frequency – and the country of origin of the above policy leads the world in this domain – we need a cultural shift towards the fostering of the positive inner life force of all men, especially the young. The salutogenic dynamic in the individual, his/her capacity to manage the environment, is a personal/spiritual dimension to be fostered, as we have indicated. Just as the individual child's – in this case boy child's – inner force needs positive reinforcement, so does the collective boy child and young man, as it were. Our society needs to be saying to boys and young men, 'You are valued. You have a real place in our society.' In western society it is not clear that this is happening.

We have said that a balanced health approach must include planning for requisite treatment and appropriate care for the population(s) in question. One of the slogans of the 'Health for All'/Primary Health Care approach was that health care should manifest the 'three A's': it should be *affordable, accessible and (culturally) appropriate.*

As regards men, I deal here only with the 'accessible and the culturally appropriate', leaving the 'affordable' to the discussion on equity below. As has been said, it is commonplace to hear, in western societies at least, that men do not use health services enough, that they are reluctant to seek help for more physical ailments and, with regard to their mental health, reluctant to get in touch with their feelings – echoes, again, of a deficit view of men. A salutogenic approach would challenge this and acknowledge the salutogenic impulse that is in men. Our thinking around 'boys' and men's health' would start from the acknowledgement of the positive life force, the salutogenic drive in boys and men, sometimes manifesting itself differently from girls and women, of course. Again, the model of the nourishing family comes to mind: we foster the energy of girls and boys, while accepting that this energy may manifest itself differently in both. We should also avoid stereotyping here; sure, there are gender differences, but there is no female monopoly of gentleness and thoughtfulness, just as there is no male monopoly of energetic drive. Maleness, in a salutogenic perspective, would not be something to be apologized for and 'controlled', but honoured and encouraged in positive ways. In the Australian context, before blaming men for too much risk taking, society should celebrate the useful risk taking men get involved in for the benefit of society as a whole. Those of us who depend on volunteer firemen (99 per cent of fire-fighting volunteers are men) to preserve their lives and homes and health should have no difficulty in beginning from the positive.

As for men's use of health services, a salutogenic approach would be to ask: to what extent are these services 'male-friendly'? Can such an exhortation be necessary when many of the prestigious positions in health systems are held by men, or at least men from a certain class? As Richard Fletcher has pointed out many times, the fact that, as women began to point out several decades ago, health services do not always meet women's needs does not allow one to come to the conclusion that these services are meeting men's needs (Fletcher et al, 2002).

Because of the child-nurturing role women have in many societies, many women have learned to negotiate the space between society and the medical profession in ways men have not. In western society, much of the energy of the health services is geared towards women, especially in the context of their reproductive functions. We notice this particularly when Third World countries have their health policies dictated to them by western institutions and 'donors': there is not just a lack of a systems view of the needs of the whole population (which would include men as one group to be 'cared' for), often even the focus on women sees them mainly as mothers, and men as such often do not feature at all. It is important to have health services that see women in wider perspectives than their nurturing role, but it is also important to ask if the services are doing what they can to make themselves more accessible to men.

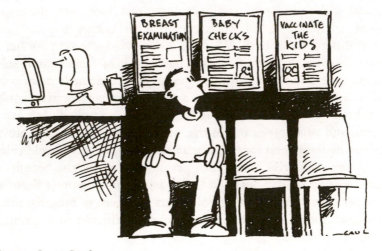

Source: Greg Gaul
Man in the waiting room

SOCIAL DETERMINANTS OF HEALTH/CREATION OF SALUTOGENIC ENVIRONMENTS: THE CASE OF MEN

A major characteristic of the expanded vision of health that has been described earlier, as regards society, is that it should adopt a social, systemic view of health, including the biological but encompassing consideration of the social determinants of health. The perspective coming from the work on the social determinants of health, taken in conjunction with what we have called the creation of salutogenic environments, can free much western thinking and planning for men's health from existing limiting mindsets.

This inclusion of the social determinants of health would mean widening the perspective, for example, of the Doctors' Reform Society and its clones, to create a mindset that looks to see what can be done about creating environments that are genuinely concerned with fostering boys' and men's health. Even if one were simply to take the list of determinants of health suggested by the WHO in its booklet already mentioned, *Social Determinants of Health: The Solid Facts* (Wilkinson and Marmot, 2003), and applied them to men, one might have the outlines of a men's *health* policy rather than a medically driven disease policy or a psychopathology-driven one focusing on men's violence. In a men's health policy, the acknowledgement of the impact of the social determinants of health would mean an acceptance of the fact that there are serious factors impacting on the life of men that lie beyond their control: more visits to the doctor and more exercise and less alcohol, on their own, will not guarantee better health. The perspective of social determinants of health imposes humility and respect on the part of policy-makers and providers. Some of the social determinants suggested by *The Solid Facts* are considered in the following paragraphs.

The social gradient

Most diseases and causes of death are more common lower down the social hierarchy. The social gradient in health reflects material disadvantage and the effects of insecurity, anxiety and lack of social integration.
                                    Wilkinson and Marmot (2003), p7

This reminds us to acknowledge that men are not a homogenous bundle and that social stratification is still a major factor influencing health, including men's health. Those who use the *Titanic* as an analogy of social life – upper, middle and lower classes with stratified access to lifeboats – are offering us a useful image, but they should not forget those who are below even the third-class passengers, those who stoked the boilers in the bowels of the ship and who perished as a result: all of them men. Simplified versions of *patriarchy*, like all salvation stories, are far from doing justice to the complexities of life and health.

Stress

> *Social and psychological circumstances can cause long-term stress. Continuing anxiety, insecurity, low self-esteem, social isolation and lack of control over work and home life have powerful effects on health. Such psychosocial risks accumulate during life and increase the chances of poor mental health and premature death. Long periods of anxiety and insecurity and the lack of supportive friendships are damaging in whatever area of life they arise.*
>
> Wilkinson and Marmot (2003), p8

To suggest that there needs to be an acknowledgement of the role of stress in understanding men's health is not to suggest that women live stress-free lives. Rather, it is to point to the fact that stress is often experienced and dealt with differently by men and women. The role of stress in men's health profiles is increasingly recognized. Expectations on boys and men, whether social or economic, can be the cause of great stress. For example, in a world of shifting job opportunities, the notion of permanent employment may well be a thing of the past. Yet, despite the discourse about the importance of men not identifying themselves too closely with their occupation, many men both see themselves and are seen by their families as the main providers, responsible for the delivery of the basic necessities of life. Permanent insecurity of job tenure in such a context is a recipe for constant stress.

Early life

The nurturing all children can be seen to be the encouragement of their own salutogenic drive, their life force. We need to build salutogenic environments for them and the resilience required to deal with the challenges life will present them with. In the case of boys a salutogenic perspective leads us to question a certain pathologizing which can be observed, for example, in the diagnosis of attention deficiency hyperactivity disorder (ADHD). One can either unquestioningly accept that many children, overwhelmingly boys, have a chemical imbalance which leads to behavioural 'abnormalities' and needs to be regulated through medication, or one can look to a wider explanation of this phenomenon. Or else one can ask the question: is this a classic case of the medicalization of a social phenomenon? Are we witnessing and sometimes colluding with a harmful pathologizing of boys (de Grandpre, 1999).

Social exclusion/social support

Men and boys may have different ways from women of expressing their social nature and their need for contact with others, but connectedness and social support are as important for them as for women. In one study of older men, a respondent said that when he came to his group of supportive 'mates' he didn't feel 'like a load of old rubbish'; like most people he needed some form of validation from others and he found it with a group of his peers, in an organized group of older men set up and run by themselves to meet just such a need (Macdonald et al, 2000). In many societies, after retirement or especially retrenchment, men experience that they are not valued, and what this older man was saying was that his group offered him positive affirmation of himself. He wouldn't have used the words, but the group can be seen to be offering him a salutogenic environment. It offered him a place for his own energies to engage with others and to be supported by them. In most societies men see an important part of their self-worth as being related to their employment status. One can challenge the 'construction of masculinity' which brings this about, but a more positive (and health) orientation would be provided by a salutogenic framework which would acknowledge the contribution men make to society and their families and offer supportive environments to men whose job security is threatened or taken away.

Men's use or non-use of health services

The social determinants of health/salutogenic approach is again a useful outlook here when, in this context, one is faced again with deficit stereotypes about men: 'They do not access mental health services because they do not get in touch with their feelings' is one of the mantras of many health professionals faced by the non-engagement of their services with their male populations. A non-deficit approach would not start from this deficit view. It would be concerned with encouraging a salutogenic orientation in each individual and in creating environments supportive of their health – in this case access to health services – in ways appropriate and attractive to men. The question should not be how we can adapt men to the service, for example by 'deconstructing their masculinity' or destroying a culture of 'hegemonic masculinity', as has frequently been suggested (see, for example, Lee and Owens, 2002). We should be asking: How can we ensure that the service is adapted to men and their needs? An evaluation of a phone-in service for people in stress and at risk of suicide recognized the underutilization by men. At first the by now standard 'explanations' were offered: men's reluctance to divulge their innermost thoughts, etc. The manager of this service, a woman, questioned this direction. Her approach was rather: if we have a service aimed at men and they do not use it, it may be of limited use to seek to adapt the user to the service, rather it makes sense to see how we adapt the service to men. Because women will more often use general counselling services and because more counsellors are women, the service may become sensitized to women's particular needs. This shift in perspective brought about a more man-friendly approach, involving a 'task-oriented' approach to counselling. And the result? Greater call-back by men (Bender, psychologist, personal communication, 2004).

We have already suggested that much of what passes for 'evidence' in the matter of men's health is, to say the least, somewhat limited. In the case of the Doctors' Reform Society and other men's health initiatives, many policies seem to have been shaped by those who have been dealing with the victims of abuse. All violence, including male violence, needs to be dealt with by society at large and health systems as well, but cannot be the main grounding for a rational health system for one major sub-group of the population. In their position paper of 2002, 'World report on violence and health', the WHO offers us a framework for understanding and dealing with all kinds of violence. They suggest an ecological perspective, of the kind already mentioned in the chapter on the social determinants of health, and go on to say that one of the four main steps in dealing in a scientific way with violence as a public health issue involves:

> *Investigating why violence occurs – that is, conducting research to determine:*
>
> - *the causes and correlates of violence;*
> - *the factors that increase or decrease the risk for violence;*
> - *the factors that might be modifiable through interventions …*
>
> *Public health is above all characterized by its emphasis on prevention. Rather than simply accepting or reacting to violence, its starting point is the strong conviction that violent behaviour and its consequences can be prevented.*
>
> WHO (2002b), p3

All this is consistent with what has been called in this work a salutogenic approach to health systems.

OTHER SECTORS AND MEN'S HEALTH

To continue the application of a salutogenic health approach to men's health, we should turn to the incorporation of the elements of the WHO's Health for All perspectives. The first of these is what the WHO calls intersectoral collaboration, the acknowledgement of the contribution to the maintenance of health of both individuals and communities, of non-medical sectors, salutogenic environments, and, of course, the inverse, the creation of pathogenic environments. Once this role has been accepted, it is obvious that it should lead to action: a salutogenic health approach to men's health means planning with other sectors to prevent harm and to promote the health of this part of the population.

An obvious example of a sector whose role should be incorporated into health planning would be the education sector. The impact of school on all children's lives is considerable and in the case of boy's mental health and well-being calls for some close consideration. A good illustration of the significance of the axis school–health service–home in the matter of boy's health is the issue of the diagnosis of attention deficiency disorder (ADD) and the related attention deficiency hyperactivity disorder (ADHD), which we have already mentioned. It is an example of the need for a cultural shift in the way some western societies view maleness. A salutogenic approach would challenge this and seek to validate the role of boys and their energy.

The work of Professor Faith Trent and her colleagues on the experience of boys' schools is revealing here. In a study across the public and private sectors they found that the overwhelming experience of many of these boys was that they did not find themselves respected in schools (Trent and Slade, 2000). If there is an 'issue' about boys in schools, and there clearly is, it is interesting to note the parallel with the 'issue' of men and health services. In both cases there is a mismatch, something which does not fit. In both cases the service adopts an explanatory framework which sees the problem as lying in the client. The explanation is that 'there is something wrong with them' rather than looking to what might be deficient in the service. A salutogenic preoccupation would be looking to foster the capacity of boys to deal with the environment, but it would also be actively seeking to ensure that the environment, in this case the school environment, was a place where boys felt they were clearly respected.

The ease with which psychopathology is invoked as an explanation for what is happening here is alarming. One can empathize with the overworked and under-resourced teacher facing crowded classrooms with boys being asked to remain seated and focused for hours at a time. One can empathize with the nuclear family, or the single-parent family dealing with boys' energies in addition to the 'usual' stress of child rearing. No matter how guarded the school interaction with the home may be, there is often the implication that the family is at fault, and sometimes challenging both the school and the medical profession in their diagnosis of this 'condition' can be very awkward for the family.

It is heartening to note that there are serious voices raised with what could be called a more salutogenic approach to the whole issue of what is, after all, largely a behavioural and not a medical issue.

EQUITY AND MEN'S HEALTH

The Health for All initiative made an appeal for equity to be considered as an essential dimension of health planning, and the social determinants of health literature is generally part of a wider debate on inequalities in health. It should go without saying that improvements in the social conditions of society at large will benefit all citizens, including men. Men in poorer social economic situations die younger than those further up the social gradient. The discrimination suffered by black working-class men in societies where they are in the minority means that they suffer more than others.

PARTICIPATION

The call for greater participation was part of the original Health for All strategy and at the very least this should mean structured efforts to incorporate populations' perspectives in health planning. As regards men's health there is little evidence of such 'participatory planning'.

MEN BEHAVING BADLY

We have said that all western health systems focus on the pathological. Usually the emphasis is on biological pathologies. In the case of men's health, at least, this has flowed into social pathologies rather easily: men as perpetrators, men as abusers, men as violent.

If we want a concern for men's health which, *inter alia*, helps us create a positive identity for the coming generations of men as well as offering a framework for positive health for the present generation, then we have to find a way to speak about men and masculinity that doesn't subscribe to these pathologizing narratives. There is a need to put things in balance, to adopt a salutogenic approach to men's health. This will mean a focus on *health* and the individual's and community's capacity to interact with their total environment as well as the concern to create environments that are salutogenic in that they foster boys' and men's well-being. There is need for a mindset that counters the medical concern with the pathological with a salutogenic vision of populations, be it adolescents, older people, or in this instance, men.

In some societies, as in Australia, we may find in the indigenous culture a 'talk to talk and a walk to walk' – a way of thinking and doing health and health care. It is ironic that we should look to the indigenous community for direction since it is a community which has been largely decimated by the white colonizing experience (see, for example, Human Rights and Equal Opportunities Commission, 1997). Without in any way colonizing the aboriginal men's health movement, we suggest that we can find in it a way forward, to build a new language of men's health. We can build a language of 'men's business' in health, a language which is respectful of 'women's business', but claims, without any need for aggression, the right to talk of men's health as something complementary to women's health – a talk, or discourse, which is ready to address contradictions but from the outset and throughout is based on the foundation that being male is what we are and it is good. There is an inbuilt salutogenic approach to the Australian indigenous understanding of health which could benefit the larger society.

CONCLUSION

This book is about the way we think about health and the way we organize health services. It suggests that we really have no excuse for not rethinking health in ways that correspond better to what we are learning about some of health's complexities and the importance of context. Specifically, I suggest that present dominant ways of thinking and doing do not sufficiently respect, in general, the agency of the person and their interaction with their environment. The book presents the idea – not new to many cultures and even to parts of the globalized western culture – that health is the dynamic interaction between the life force of the person (and by extrapolation, the community) and the environment, this understood as the total biological, social, economic and political context in which people live out their lives. The global popular and professional 'health' culture is often focused on the pathological and *pathogenic*. In this book the notion of *salutogenic* is borrowed from Antonovsky as a way of moving towards thinking and doing health rather than focusing narrowly on disease and the pathological. I expand the notion of 'salutogenic' to include those parts of the environment which, when encountered by our life force, can nourish it and our responsibility to make our social, cultural, economic and political environments as health-enhancing as possible: that is what I mean by salutogenic environments. Although I never met Antonovsky, an Israeli scholar, my Palestinian colleague, Professor Rita Giacaman, introduced me to his widow in Jerusalem in the early 1990s. Mrs Antonovsky assured me that my expanded use of the expression was consistent with his thoughts.

The chapter on men's health is simply an illustration of how such thinking can lead us towards what I feel will be more fruitful ways for society, health services and the health of this particular sub-population. The same approach, of course, needs to be applied to other groups and sub-populations. But that is, as they say, another story, or several other books.

REFERENCES

Antonovsky, A. (1979) *Health, Stress and Coping*, Jossey-Bass, San Francisco

Antonovsky, A. (1987) *Unravelling the Mystery of Health: How People Manage Stress and Stay Well*, Jossey-Bass, San Francisco

Australian Bureau of Statistics (2003) 'Australian social trends, 2002: Health, mortality and morbidity: Mortality of Aboriginal and Torres Strait Islander Peoples', available at www.abs.gov.au/Ausstats/abs%40. nsf/94713ad445ff1425ca25682000192af2/cd784ff808c14658ca256bcd 008272f6!OpenDocument

Australian Government, Department of Health and Ageing (2004) 'National comorbidity project', available at www.health.gov.au/internet/wcms/Publishing.nsf/Content/health-pubhlth-strateg-comorbidity-index.htm

Barrow, J. (2004) 'Free care for elderly is sensible, necessary and affordable', *The Scotsman*, available at http://thescotsman.scotsman.com/ opinion.cfm?id=912032004

Baur, C. (2001) personal communication

Bender, C. Psychologists (2004) personal communication, 22 November

Bengel, J., Strittmatter, R. and Willmann, H. (1999) 'What keeps people healthy? The current state of discussion and the relevance of Antonovsky's salutogenic model of health', *Research and Practice of Health Promotion, volume 4*, Federal Centre for Health Education, Cologne

Berkman, L. F. and Glass, T. (2000) 'Social integration, social networks, social support, and health', in Berkman, L. F. and Kawachi, I. (eds) *Social Epidemiology*, Oxford University Press, New York, pp137–173

Berkman, L. F. and Kawachi, I. (eds) (2000) *Social Epidemiology*, Oxford University Press, New York, Oxford

Blane, D., White, I. and Morriss, J. (1995) 'Education, social circumstances and mortality', in Blane, D., Brunner, E. J. and Wilkinson, R. (eds) *Health and Social Organization*, London, Routledge

Brown, D. (2004) 'Report on overseas study visit to England and France', April 2004, available at www.parliament.sa.gov.au/catalog/travel reports/2004/20047230935.pdf

Brunner, E. J. (2000) 'Towards a new social biology', in Berkman, L. F. and Kawachi, I. (eds) *Social Epidemiology*, Oxford University Press, New York, Oxford

Caldicott, F., Barchard, C., Haldane, J., Hornby, S., McGuffin, P., Pleming, N., Richards, M., Taylor, P., Wilkie, A. and Young, S. (1998) *Mental Disorders And Genetics: The Ethical Context*, Nuffield Council on Bioethics, London, accessed 2004 at www.nuffieldbioethics.org/file Library/pdf/mentaldisorders2001.pdf

Canada Health Network (2004) 'What makes people healthy?', accessed 2004 at www.canadian-health-network.ca/servlet/ContentServer?cid=1005630&pagename=CHNRCS%2FCHNResource%2FFAQCHN·ResourceTemplate&lang=En&c=CHNResource

Cannon, W. B. (1932) *The Wisdom of the Body*, WW Norton & Co, New York

Chapman, S. (2003) 'Reducing tobacco consumption', *N.S.W. Public Health Bulletin*, 14(3), 46–48

Cobb, S. (1975) 'Social support as a moderator of life stress', *Psychosomatic Med*, 38, 300–313

Cohen, N. (2004) 'Comment', *The Observer*, London, 28 March, p29

Cohen, S., Doyle, W. J., Skoner, D. P., Rabin, B. S. and Gwaltney, J. M., Jr (1997) 'Social ties and susceptibility to the common cold', *JAMA*, 277, 1940–1944

Council of Social Services NSW (NCOSS) (2000) 'Savings from short hospital stays need re-investing in the community', in *Earlier Discharge* (report compiled by the NCOSS and NSW Community Health Association), accessed 2004 at www.ncoss.org.au/media/archive/health.html#16.10.00

Crenson, M. (2000) accessed 2004 at www.nandotimes.com/24hour/modbee/healthscience/story/0,1655,500221378-500316259-501774250-0,00.html

De Grandpre, R. (1999) *Ritalin Nation: Rapid-fire Culture and the Transformation of Human Consciousness*, WW Norton, New York

Devanesen, D. (2000) 'Traditional Aboriginal medicine practice in the Northern Territory', paper presented at the International Symposium on Traditional Medicine, Kobe, Japan, accessed 2004 at www.nt.gov.au/health/comm_health/abhealth_strategy/Traditional%20Aboriginal%20Medicine%20-%20Japan%20Paper.pdf

Development Dialogue (1972) Dag Hammarskjold Foundation, Ovre Slottsgatan 2, SE-753 10, Uppsala, Sweden

De Voe, J. (2003) 'A policy transformed by politics: the case of the 1973 Australian Community Health Program', *Journal of Health Politics, Policy and Law*, 28(1), 77–108

Doctor's Reform Society Policy Statements (undated) Australia, accessed at www.drs.org.au/policies/policy08.htm

Donelan, K., Blendon, R. J., Schoen, C., Davis, K. and Binns, K. (1999) 'The cost of health system change: Public discontent in five nations', *Health Affairs*, May/June, 18(3), 206–216, accessed 2004 at http://content.healthaffairs.org/cgi/search?qbe=healthaff;23/3/119&journalcode=healthaff&minscore=5000

Donovan, A. (2004) *Buddha Da*, Cannongate Books, Edinburgh

Doyal, L. (1979) *The Political Economy of Health*, Pluto Press, London

Dubos, R. (1970) *Man, Medicine, and Environment*, Pelican, Harmondsworth

Ernst, E. (2000) 'The role of complementary and alternative medicine', *British Medical Journal*, 321, 1133–1135

Evans, R. G., Hodge, M. and Pless, I. B. (1994) 'If not genetics, then what?', in Evans, R. G., Bartrer, M. L. and Marmor, T. R. (eds) *Why Are Some People Healthy and Others Not*, Aldine de Gruyter, New York

Evans, R. G., Marmor, T. R. and Barer, L. M. (eds) (1994) *Why Are Some People Healthy and Others Not? The Determinants of Health of Populations*, A de Gruyter, New York

Fanon, F. (1968) *Black Skin, White Masks* (1st edn), Grove Press, New York

Fletcher, R., Higginbotham, N. and Dobson, A. (2002) 'Men's perceived health needs', *Journal of Health Psychology*, 7(3), 233–241

Focosi, D. (2001) 'Intrinsic aetiology', accessed 2004 at http://focosi.altervista.org/intrinsicaetiology.htm

Garmezy, N. and Rutter, M. (1983) *Stress, Coping and Development in Children*, McGraw-Hill, New York

Garmezy, N., Masters, A. and Tellegen, A. (1984) 'The study of stress and competence in children: A building block for developmental psychopathology', *Child Development*, 55, 97–111

Garrett, L. (2000) *Betrayal of Trust, The Collapse of Global Public Health*, Hyperion, New York

Glaser, R., Kiecolt-Glaser, J. K., Speicher, C. E. et al (1985) 'Stress loneliness and changes in herpesvirus latency', *Journal of Behavioral Medicine*, 8, 249–260.

Graham, H. (1986) 'Women smoking and family health', paper presented at the British Sociological Association Medical Sociology Group Conference, September, New York

Grzywacz, J. G. and Fuqua, J. (2000) 'The social ecology of health: Leverage points and linkages', *Behavioural Medicine*, Fall, accessed 2004 at www.findarticles.com/p/articles/mi_m0GDQ/is_3_26/ai_90304031

Hamrell, S. and Nordberg, O. (1972–1984) *Development Dialogue*, Dag Hammarskjold Foundation, Uppsala

Hauser, S. T., Vieyra, M. A. B., Jacobson, A. M. and Wertlieb, D. (1989) 'Family aspects of vulnerability and resilience in adolescence: A theoretical perspective', in Dugan, T. F. and Coles, R. (eds) *The Child in our Times, Studies in the Development of Resiliency*, Brunel Mazel, New York

Health Canada, 'Population Health', accessed 2004 at www.hc-sc.gc.ca/hppb/phdd/approach/index.html

Human Rights and Equal Opportunity Commission (1997) *Bringing Them Home, A Guide to the Findings and Recommendations of the National Inquiry into the Separation of Aboriginal and Torres Strait Islander Children From Their Families*, Sydney

Illich, I. (1975) *Medical Nemesis*, Caldar & Boyars, London

International Council of Nurses Fact Sheet, 'ICN on Poverty and Health: Breaking the Link', accessed 2004 at www.icn.ch/matters_poverty.htm

Jarvis, M. J. and Wardle, J. (2000) 'Social patterning of individual behaviour', in Marmot, M. and Wilkinson, R. (eds) *Social Determinants of Health*, Oxford University Press, Oxford

Kaptchuk, T. D. (2000) *Chinese Medicine, The Web That Has No Weaver*, Random House, London

Kaptchuk, T. D. (2002) 'Acupuncture: Theory, efficacy and practice', *Annals of Internal Medicine*, 136(5), 374

Kawachi, I. and Berkman, L. (2000) 'Social cohesion, social capital, and health', in Berkman, L. and Kawachi, I. (eds) *Social Epidemiology*, Oxford University Press, New York, Oxford

Keith, A. (1919) 'The engines of the human body', lectures given at the Royal Institution of Great Britain

Kiecolt-Glaser, J., Fisher, L., Ogrocki, P., Stout, J., Speicher, C. and Glaser, R. (1987) 'Marital quality, marital disruption and immune function', *Psychosomatic Med*, 49

Kiecolt-Glaser, J., Garner, W., Speicher, C., Penn, G., Holliday, J. and Glaser, R. (1984) 'Psychosocial modifiers of immunocompetence in medical students', *Psychosomatic Med*, 46, 7–14

Kubzanski, L.D., Kawachi, I., Weiss, S. T. and Sparrow, D. (1998) 'Anxiety and coronary heart disease: A synthesis of epidemiological, psychological, and experimental evidence', *Annals of Behavioral Medicine*, 20, 47–58

Lee, C. and Owens, R. G. (2002) 'Issues for a psychology of men's health', *Journal of Health Psychology*, 7(3), 209

Levin, J. (1996) 'How religion influences morbidity and health: Reflections on natural history, salutogenesis and host resistance, *Social Science Med*, 43(5), 848–864

Levins, R. (2000) 'Is capitalism a disease? The crisis in the U.S. public health', *Monthly Review*, September

Lomas, J. and Contandriopoulos, A.P. (1994) 'Regulatory limits to medicine: Towards harmony in public- and self-regulation', in Evans, R. G., Marmor, T. R. and Barer, L. M. (eds) *Why Are Some People Healthy and Others Not? The Determinants of Health of Population*, A de Gruyter, New York

Lynch, J. and Kaplan, G. (2000) 'Socioeconomic position', in Berkman, L. F. and Kawachi, I. (eds) *Social Epidemiology*, Oxford University Press, New York, Oxford, pp13–35

Macdonald, J. (2000) *Primary Health Care*, Earthscan, London

Macdonald, J., Brown, A. and Buchanan, J. (2000) *Keeping the Balance, A Study of The Health of Older Men*, NSW Committee on Ageing

Mackenbach, J. P., Bouvier-Colle, M. H. and Jougla, E. (1990) 'Avoidable mortality and health services: A review of aggregate data studies', *Journal of Epidemiology and Community Health*, 44, 106–111

Maldonado, T. (2000) 'Factores protectores de la resiliencia en la familia, la escuela y la communidad', Conferencia Latinoamericana, *Inovaciones en Educación Médica*, Universidad Mayor de San Miguel, Cochabamba, Bolivia, 3–7 October

Marmot, M. (1996) 'The social pattern of health and disease', in Blane, D., Brunner, E. and Wilkinson, R. (eds) *Health and Social Organization: Towards a Health Policy for the 21st century*, Routledge, London

Marmot, M. (2000) 'Multi-level approaches to understanding social determinants', in Berkman, L. F. and Kawachi, I. (eds) *Social Epidemiology*, Oxford University Press, New York, Oxford

Marmot, M. and Wilkinson, R. (eds) (1999) *Social Determinants of Health*, Oxford University Press, Oxford

Marmot, M. and Wilkinson, R. (eds) (2003, (1998)) *Social Determinants of Health, The Solid Facts*, World Health Organization, Copenhagen

McCabe, D. and Holmwood, C. (2002) *Comorbidity in General Practice: The Provision of Care for People With Coexisting Mental Health Problems and Substance Use by General Practitioners* (revised report), Primary Mental Health Care Australian Resource Centre, Department of General Practice, Flinders University, Adelaide, accessed 2004 at http://som.flinders.edu.au/FUSA/PARC/comorbidityreportrevised 2002.pdf

McNeil, D. G. (2000) 'Prices for medicine are exorbitant in Africa, study says', *New York Times*, accessed 2004 at www.survivreausida.net/a4134

Menadhue, J. (2000) 'Chairman's message: Hospitals or health', *Report of the NSW Health Council: A Better Health System for NSW*, NSW Government

Monbiot, G. (2001) 'Are man-made chemicals turning against us?', *Guardian Weekly*, 11–17 January, 23, accessed 2004 at www.guardian.co.uk/GWeekly/Story/0,,420395,00.html

National Health Debate and Poll, accessed 2004 at www.youdebate.com/ DEBATES/national_health_care.HTM

National Health Service (England) (2000) 'Meeting the challenge: a strategy for the allied health professions', accessed at www.dh.gov.uk/asset Root/04/05/51/80/04055180.pdf

Navarro, V. (1986) *Crisis, Health, and Medicine: A Social Critique*, Tavistock Publications, New York, London

New Health Digest (2004) 'Integrated health: Chinese doctors bring integrated thinking into Western practice', accessed 2004 at www.new healthdigest.com/NHDjan04/chinesemed.html

Ottawa Charter (1986) '1st International Conference on Health Promotion', accessed 2004 at www.ldb.org/iuhpe/ottawa.htm

Pankhania, J. (1994) *Liberating the National History Curriculum*, Falmer Press, London

People-to-People Health Foundation, Inc. (Project HOPE) (1999) *Health Affairs*, May/June, accessed 2004 at www.cmwf.org/publist/grants/jul99gnt.asp

Pickering, J. (2001) 'Wellbeing: The interaction between person and environment', *ESRC Seminar Series on Wellbeing: Social and Individual Determinants*, Queen Mary University of London, accessed 2004 at www2.warwick.ac.uk/fac/sci/psych/people/academic/jpickering/johnpickering/wellbeing/

Public Health Association of Australia, 'Primary Health Care', accessed at www.phaa.net.au/policy/primary.htm

Rainbow Books (1977) *Community Health: Book No. 1, General Concepts*, Health Commission of NSW

Ridley, M. (1999) *Genome, The Autobiography of a Species in 23 Chapters*, Fourth Estate, London

Rio Declaration on Environment and Development (1992) 'Agenda 21', accessed 2004 at http://habitat.igc.org/agenda21/

Ritzer, G. (2000) *The McDonaldisation of Society: New Century Edition*, Sage Publications, USA

Sapolsky, R. and Spencer, E. (1997) 'Social subordinance is associated with suppression of insulin-like growth factor I (IGF-I) in a population of wild primates', *American Journal of Physiology*, 273, R1346

Saskatchewan Public Health Association (1999) 'The link between education and health', accessed 2004 at www.cpha.ca/english/policy/pstatem/hdeterm/educa/page1.htm

Shree Gulabkunverba Ayurvedic Society (1949) *Caraka Samhita*, Jamnagar, India

Snow, J. (1855) *On the Mode of the Communication of Cholera*, accessed 2004 at www.ph.ucla.edu/epi/snow/snowbook.html

Stansfeld, S. A. (1999) 'Social support and social cohesion', in Marmot, M. and Wilkinson, R. (eds) *Social Determinants of Health*, Oxford University Press, Oxford

Stokols, D. (2000) 'Social ecology and behavioural medicine: Implications for training, practice, and policy', *Behavioural Medicine*, Fall, accessed 2004 at www.findarticles.com/p/articles/mi_m0GDQ/is_3_26/ai_90304033/print

Tarimo, E. and Creese, A. (eds) (1990) *Achieving Health For All by the Year 2000, Midway Reports of Country Experiences*, WHO, Geneva

Theorell, T. (2000) 'Working conditions and health', in Berkman, L. F. and Kawachi, I. (eds) *Social Epidemiology*, Oxford University Press, New York, Oxford, pp95–117

Thomas, P., Goodwin, J. and Goodwin, J. (1985) 'Effect of social support on stress-related changes in cholesterol levels, uric acid level and immune function in an elderly sample', *Am J Psychiatry*, 142, 735–737

Trent, F. and Slade, M. (2000) 'What the boys are saying', *International Educational Journal*, 1(3), accessed 2004 at http://ehlt.flinders.edu.au/education/iej/articles/v1n3/slade/slade.pdf

Turp, M. (2001) *Psychosomatic Health, the Body and the Word*, Palgrave, Houndmills

UNAIDS (2002) *AIDS Epidemic Update*, WHO

United Nations Second World Assembly on Ageing (2002) 'Political Declaration', Article 2, accessed 2004 at www.un.org/ageing/coverage/declaration.htm

Unschuld, P. U. (1985) *Medicine in China, A History of Ideas*, University of California Press, Berkeley

Vinson, T. (1999) 'Unequal in life: The distribution of social disadvantage in Victoria and New South Wales'

Virchow, R. (1859) 'Industrialisation and the sanitary movement', in Rosen, G. (ed.) *Virchow*, accessed 2004 at www.pathguy.com/lectures/virchow.htm

Walsh, J. A. and Warren, K. S. (1979) 'Selective primary health care: An interim strategy for disease control in developing countries', *Social Science and Medicine*, 14C, 145–163, reprinted from *New England Journal of Medicine*, 301

Walton, H. J. (1983) 'The place of primary health care in medical education in the UK: A survey', *Medical Education*, 17, 141–147

Walton, H. J. (1985) 'Primary health care in European medical education: A survey', *Medical Education*, 19, 167–188

Warner, E. E. and Smith, R. S. (1982) *Vulnerable but Invincible: A Study of Resilient Children*, McGraw-Hill, New York

Watt, G., Professor of General Practice, University of Glasgow, personal communication, April 2001

Weil, A. (1996) *Health and Healing*, Warner Books, London

Werner, D. and Sanders, D. (1997) *Questioning the Solution: The Politics of Primary Health Care and Child Survival with an In-depth critique of Oral Rehydration Therapy*, Health Wrights

White, M. (1995) *Re-authoring Lives: Interviews and Essays*, Dulwich Centre Publications, Adelaide, South Australia

Wilkinson, R. G. (1999) 'Prosperity, redistribution, health and welfare', in Marmot, M. and Wilkinson, R. G. (eds) *Social Determinants of Health*, Oxford University Press, Oxford

Wilkinson, R. (2000) Concluding presentation, 12th National Health Promotion Conference, Melbourne, Australia, 1 November

Wilkinson, R. G. and Marmot, M. (eds) (1998) *Social Determinants of Health: The Solid Facts*, World Health Organization, Copenhagen

Williams, S. J. (2003) 'Marrying the social and the biological: A rejoinder to Newton', *The Sociological Review*

Wisner, B. (1988) *Power and Need in Africa: Basic Human Needs and Development Policies*, Earthscan, London

World Bank (1993) *World Development Report*, Oxford University Press, New York

World Health Organization (undated) 'Ageing and Life Course Program', accessed 2004 at www.who.int/hpr/ageing/index.htm

World Health Organization (1978) International Conference on Primary Health Care (Alma Atu), WHO/Unicef, Geneva

World Health Organization (2001) 'WHO Global Strategy for Containment of Antimicrobial Resistance', accessed 2004 at www.who.int/csr/resources/publications/drugresist/en/EGlobal_Strat.pdf

World Health Organization (2002a) 'Active Ageing: Policy Framework', WHO, accessed 2004 at www.who.int/hpr/ageing/ActiveAgeingPolicy Frame.pdf

World Health Organization (2002b) 'World report on violence and health', accessed 2004 at www.who.int/violence_injury_prevention/violence/world_report/en/full_en.pdf

World Health Organization (2003) 'Index of vaccines', accessed 2004 at www.who.int/vaccines-documents/DocsPDF02

World Health Organization (2004a) 'The World Health Report', Chapter 3, accessed 2004 at www.who.int/whr/2004/chapter3/en/index1.html

World Health Organization (2004b) 'The Right to Water', Chapter 1, accessed 2004 at www.who.int/water_sanitation_health/rightowater/en/print.html

Index